Pre-Clinical
Conservative
Dentistry
SECOND EDITION

Pre-Clinical
Conservative
Dentistry

SECOND EDITION

Vimal K Sikri

MDS, DOOP (PU), DEME (AIU), FICD

Professor and Head
Department of Conservative Dentistry and Endodontics
and
Principal
Punjab Government Dental College and Hospital
Amritsar, Punjab

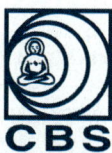

CBS

CBS Publishers & Distributors Pvt Ltd

New Delhi • Bengaluru • Chennai • Kochi • Kolkata • Mumbai
Bhopal • Bhubaneswar • Hyderabad • Jharkhand • Nagpur • Patna • Pune • Uttarakhand • Dhaka (Bangladesh)

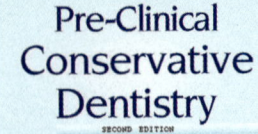

ISBN: 978-81-239-2496-0

Second Edition: 2015
Reprint: 2019

First Edition: 2009

Published by Satish Kumar Jain and produced by Varun Jain for

CBS Publishers & Distributors Pvt Ltd

4819/XI Prahlad Street, 24 Ansari Road, Daryaganj, New Delhi 110 002, India.

Ph: 23289259, 23266861, 23266867   Fax: 011-23243014   Website: www.cbspd.com
e-mail: delhi@cbspd.com; cbspubs@airtelmail.in

Corporate Office: 204 FIE, Industrial Area, Patparganj, Delhi 110 092
Ph: 4934 4934   Fax: 4934 4935   e-mail: publishing@cbspd.com; publicity@cbspd.com

Branches

- **Bengaluru:** Seema House 2975, 17th Cross, K.R. Road,
  Banasankari 2nd Stage, Bengaluru 560 070, Karnataka
  Ph: +91-80-26771678/79   Fax: +91-80-26771680   e-mail: bangalore@cbspd.com
- **Chennai:** 7, Subbaraya Street, Shenoy Nagar, Chennai 600 030, Tamil Nadu
  Ph: +91-44-26680620, 26681266   Fax: +91-44-42032115   e-mail: chennai@cbspd.com
- **Kochi:** 42/1325, 1326, Power House Road, Opposite KSEB Power House,
  Ernakulam 682 018, Kochi, Kerala
  Ph: +91-484-4059061-65   Fax: +91-484-4059065   e-mail: kochi@cbspd.com
- **Kolkata:** 6/B, Ground Floor, Rameswar Shaw Road, Kolkata-700 014, West Bengal
  Ph: +91-33-22891126, 22891127, 22891128   e-mail: kolkata@cbspd.com
- **Mumbai:** 83-C, Dr E Moses Road, Worli, Mumbai-400018, Maharashtra
  Ph: +91-22-24902340/41   Fax: +91-22-24902342   e-mail: mumbai@cbspd.com

Representatives

• **Bhopal**	0-8319310552	• **Bhubaneswar**	0-9911037372	• **Hyderabad**	0-9885175004	• **Jharkhand**	0-9811541605
• **Nagpur**	0-9021734563	• **Patna**	0-9334159340	• **Pune**	0-9623451994	• **Uttarakhand**	0-9716462459
• **Dhaka (Bangladesh)**	01912-003485						

Printed at : Rashtriya Printers, Dilshad Garden, Delhi, India

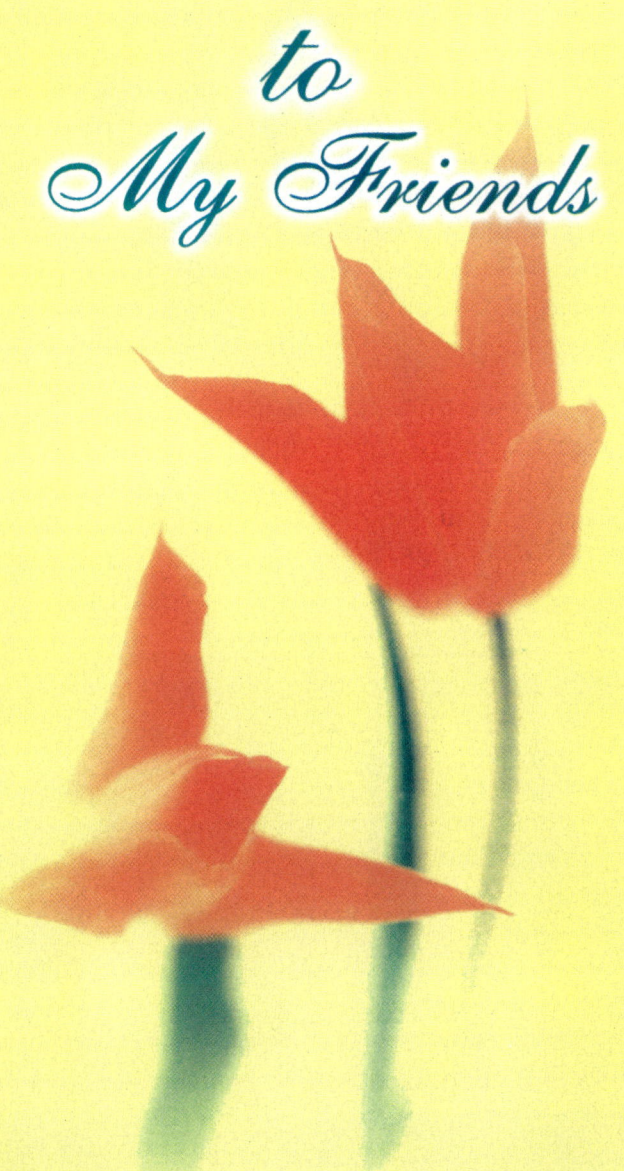

to
My Friends

Friendship is intelligence above language:
No words, only meaning

Preface to the Second Edition

The criticism and/or praise are considered 'noble' only where the critic is not a 'rival'. Since I could not find any rival in my career, I took it positively listening to all praises/criticism of my dear colleagues, friends, teachers and students.

The outcome of all this is in your hands in the form of revised and improved second edition of *Pre-Clinical Conservative Dentistry*. The pre-clinical training is important for budding dentists since it is to be carried to the clinics working on patients.

The text has been revised and simplified using lucid language. New line diagrams and photographs have been added to understand the operative procedures easily. The tables and boxes are also modified to highlight the important points for the young readers. The glossary at the end will provide an opportunity for the students to revise the text and prepare for *viva voce* examination. I hope the book will be a boon for students, teachers and anyone interested in learning and teaching conservative dentistry.

I am wholeheartedly grateful to my students, Shaveta Seth, Meghna Mittal, Shikha Sharma and Priyanka Setia, for checking and rechecking the manuscript and the diagrams as well. My sincere thanks to Mr Sunny for creating nice line diagrams in CorelDRAW.

My dear wife Poonam, my sons Ankit and Arpit, and daughter Annupriya, deserve special thanks since they always bear my 'lost in thinking' attitude. Their motivation is commendable and visible in the text.

Once again, I will request my dear students and the teachers as well to read the book thoroughly and suggest improvements which can be incorporated in the next edition.

Vimal K Sikri

Preface to the First Edition

The operative/conservative dentistry has been considered as 'mother' of all dental subjects. The restorative skills are of utmost importance since these are the core of success in general practice. For professional training, accumulation of basic knowledge followed by acquisition of surgical skill is mandatory.

At the outset, I wish to express my sincere gratitude to Dr Vineeta Nikhil, Professor, DAV Dental College, Yamunanagar, who conceived the idea and encouraged me to write a book on *Pre-Clinical Conservative Dentistry*. The text in the book is designed for the use of students who are to enter the clinical phase of their professional course as well as practising dentists who may desire to review the operative procedures.

Extensive supervised clinical practice and chairside training is important for budding dentists to achieve excellent operative skills. Intention of the book is to make the students well versed with the basic techniques and styles of such skills. New illustrations have been planned and added to simplify the basic and the recent operative procedures. In all humility, I hope readers will find the accomplishment of these ideas in the present book, which are mandatory for the practice of dentistry.

My sincere thanks to my colleagues, Dr Renu Sroa, Dr Jagan Jyot and Dr Sangeeta Aggarwal for their cooperation and to my students, Dr Meenu, Dr Preeti, Dr Amrit, Dr Payal, Dr Gulvinder and Dr Ibadat for helping me checking the manuscript. Mr GB Singh's job is commendable, which is visible in the diagrams prepared in CorelDRAW.

Last but not the least, I am thankful to all those who contributed directly or indirectly for the better quality of the book. My dear wife, Dr Poonam and my very dear sons, Ankit and Arpit deserve special thanks, as they always stood with me in every odd hour.

Readers are the best source of inspiration. I am sincerely waiting for their suggestions and criticism so as to have a much better next edition.

Vimal K Sikri

Contents

1

Morphology of Permanent Teeth

MORPHOLOGY

Morphology is the study of form and structure. The knowledge of form of teeth is important prior to their restoration since the basic goal of restorative dentistry is to restore the tooth in such a way so as to regain the original form and shape. The exact shape and form of every surface of tooth along with the possible variations should be known to the operator before the start of cavity/tooth preparation. The students are aware of the dental anatomy by now; only to remind them, the basic features of morphology of permanent teeth are described here.

MAXILLARY TEETH

1. Central Incisor

Labial Aspect (Fig. 1.1a)

- Mesioincisal angle is slightly rounded (approximately right angle).
- Distoincisal angle is more rounded (obtuse angle).
- In males, teeth are broader with mesioincisal and distoincisal angles relatively sharp; in females, teeth are narrower with rounded mesioincisal and distoincisal angles.

Palatal Aspect (Fig. 1.1b)

- Mesial and distal sides of the crown converge lingually (palatal convergence).
- A smooth convexity called cingulum is present immediately below cervical line and is located slightly distally.

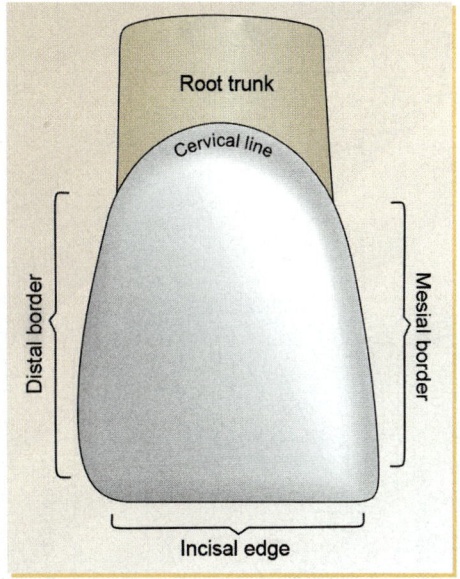

Fig. 1.1a: *Labial aspect*

- Between marginal ridges below the cingulum a shallow concavity is present known as lingual fossa (palatal fossa).
- Different shapes of lingual fossa have been recognized.

Mesial Aspect (Fig. 1.1c)

- Crown is wedge shaped or triangular with base of triangle at cervix and apex at incisal edge.
- Incisal ridge of the crown is on line with centre of root.
- Curvature of cervical line is greater on mesial surface than on distal surface.

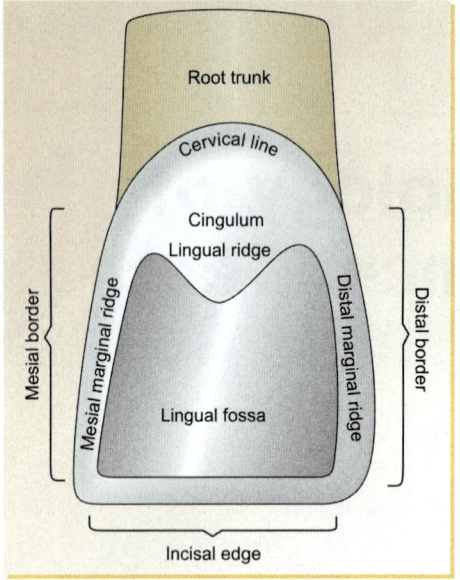

Fig. 1.1b: *Palatal aspect*

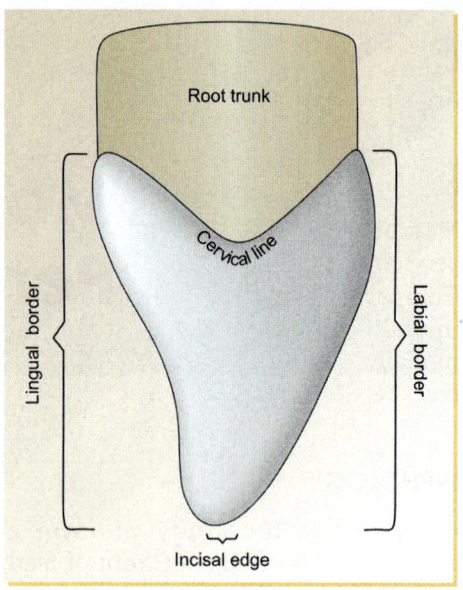

Fig. 1.1d: *Distal aspect*

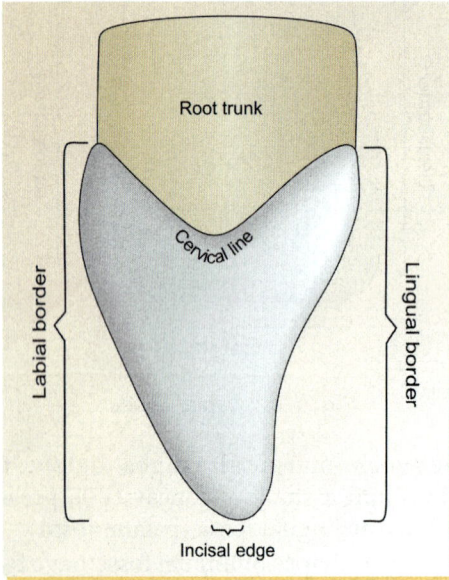

Fig. 1.1c: *Mesial aspect*

- In older adults, the incisal outline becomes flat.

Distal Aspect (Fig. 1.1d)

- Distal aspect is same as that of mesial aspect, except crown being thicker at incisal third.

- Curvature of cervical line is less than on the mesial surface.

Incisal Aspect (Fig. 1.1e)

- Lingual convergence is visible.
- Position of distoincisal angle is slightly lingual to position of mesioincisal angle (slight distolingual twist).

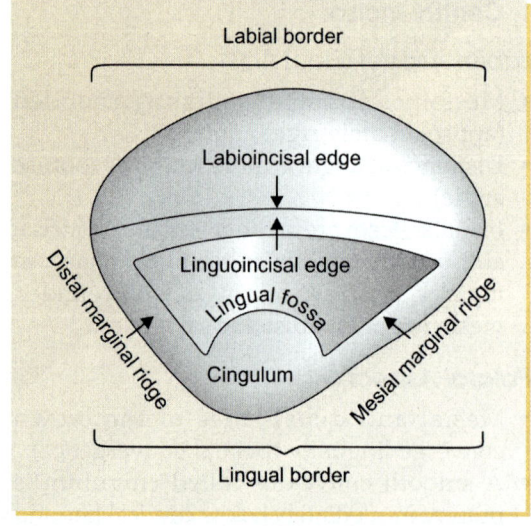

Fig. 1.1e: *Incisal aspect*

2. Lateral Incisor

It is the most frequently found missing tooth. A peg shaped (mesial and distal lobes do not develop) tooth is quite common.

Labial Aspect (Fig. 1.2a)

- Narrower mesiodistally and shorter cervicoincisally than central incisor.
- Compared to central incisor, it has rounded incisal edge and rounded incisal angles mesially and distally (mesioincisal angle 85° and distoincisal angle 95°).

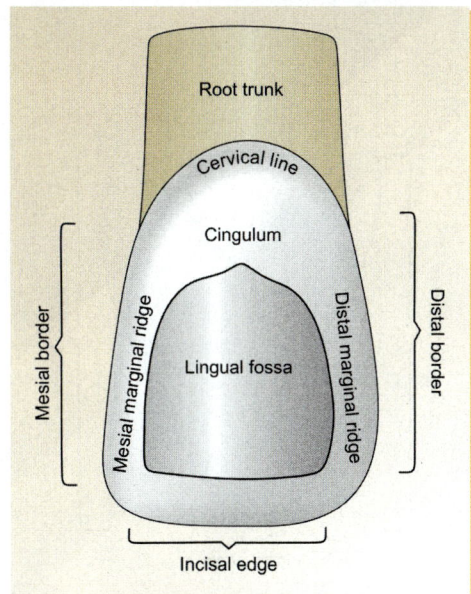

Fig. 1.2b: *Palatal aspect*

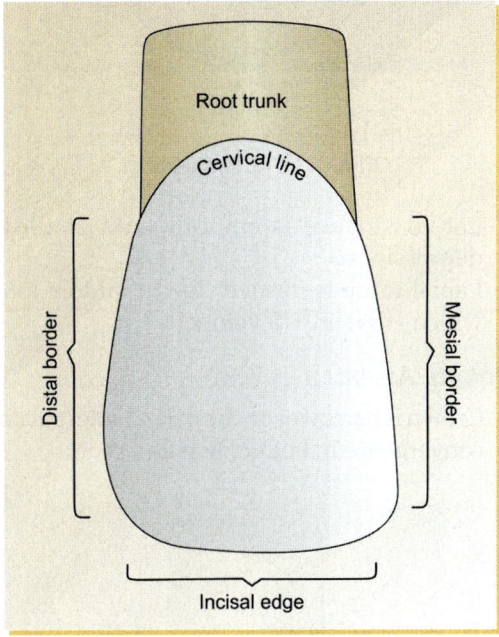

Fig. 1.2a: *Labial aspect*

Palatal Aspect (Fig. 1.2b)

- Palatal surface is narrower than labial surface.
- Marginal ridges and cingulum are more prominent than central incisor.
- There may be lingual ridges or lingual pit in the lingual fossa.

Mesial Aspect (Fig. 1.2c)

- It is triangular in shape.
- Curvature of cervical line is greater on mesial surface than on distal surface.

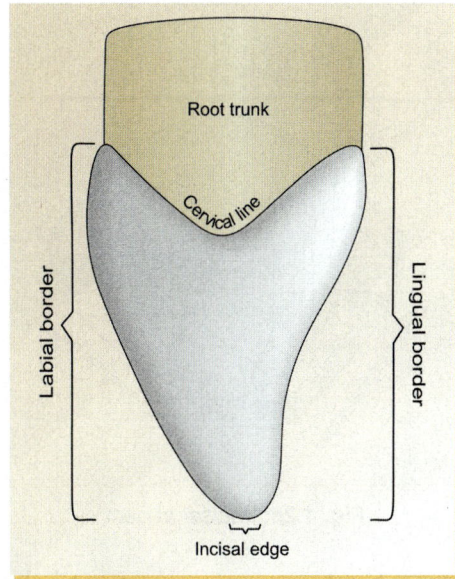

Fig. 1.2c: *Mesial aspect*

Distal Aspect (Fig. 1.2d)

- Shape is similar to that of mesial aspect.
- Curvature of cervical line is less on distal surface than on mesial surface.

Incisal Aspect (Fig. 1.2e)

- Labial margin of incisal surface is more convex than the central incisor.

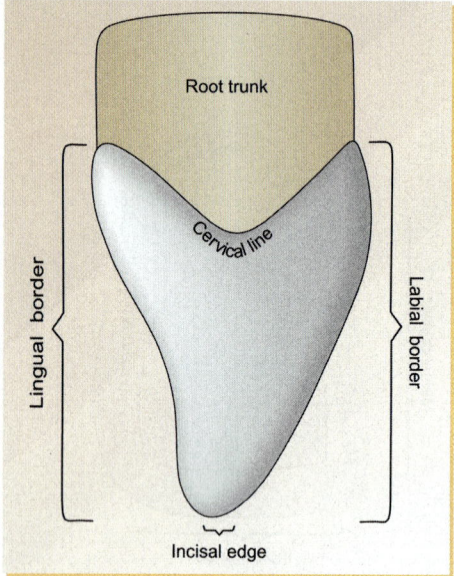

Fig. 1.2d: *Distal aspect*

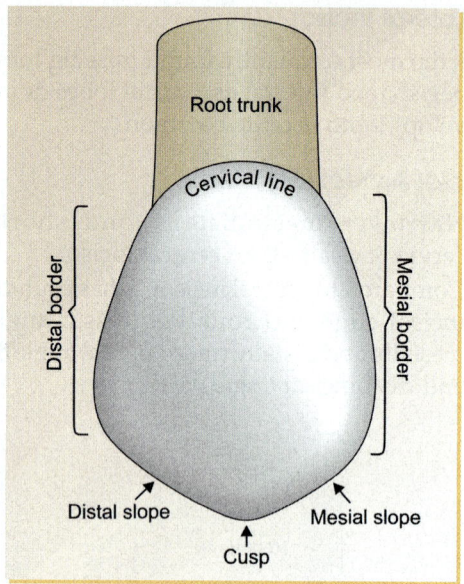

Fig. 1.3a: *Labial aspect*

- Labial surface is smooth with shallow depressions.
- Labial ridge is formed due to middle lobe which is greatly developed.

Palatal Aspect (Fig.1.3b)

- Crown is narrower on the palatal side (palatal convergence in both crown and root).

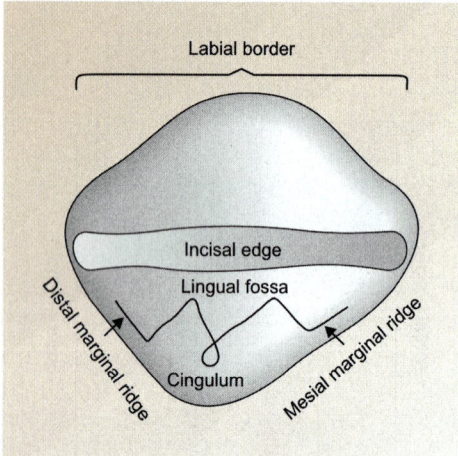

Fig. 1.2e: *Incisal aspect*

- Mesiodistal measurement is only about 0.5 mm greater than the labiolingual measurement.

3. Canine

Labial Aspect (Fig. 1.3a)

- Incisal edge comes to a distinct point, the cusp.
- Cusp has mesial slope and distal slope, mesial being shorter than the distal.

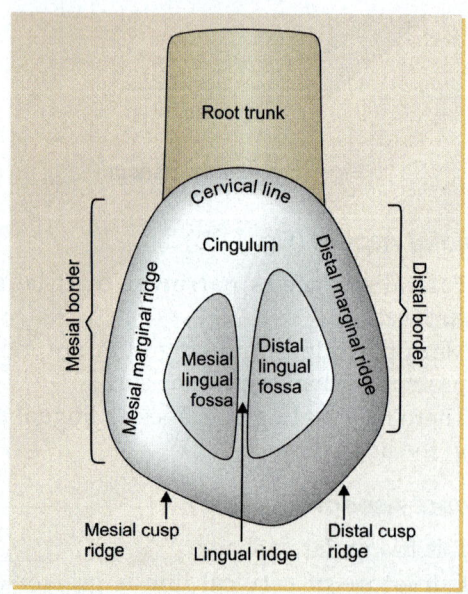

Fig. 1.3b: *Palatal aspect*

- Cingulum is large; may be pointed like a small cusp.
- There is constriction of cervix at the cemento-enamel junction. There may be a definite ridge over the cingulum known as **gingival prominence.** This prominence is present along the cervix.

Mesial Aspect (Fig.1.3c)

- Outline of crown is wedge shaped with greatest measurement being at cervical third (wedge bulkier than incisors).
- A line bisecting the cusp is labial to the line bisecting root.

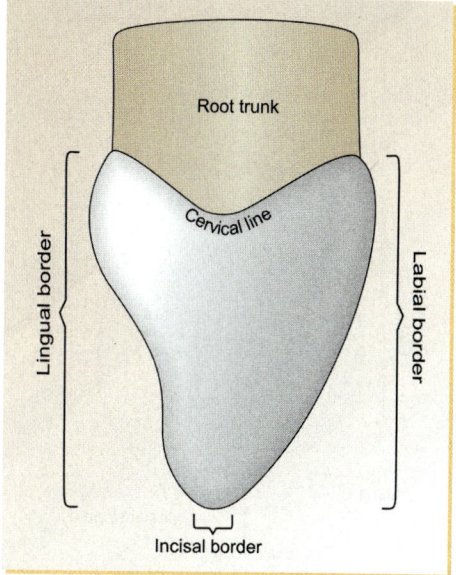

Fig. 1.3d: *Distal aspect*

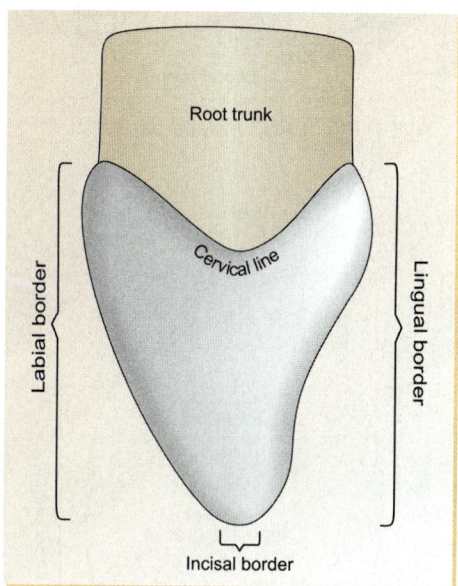

Fig. 1.3c: *Mesial aspect*

Distal Aspect (Fig. 1.3d)

Same as that of mesial aspect; however, the following variations can be seen:

- Distal marginal ridge is heavier and more irregular in outline.
- Cervical line exhibits less curvature.

Incisal Aspect (Fig. 1.3e)

- Distal cusp ridge is longer than mesial cusp ridge.
- Cingulum is located in the centre mesio-distally.

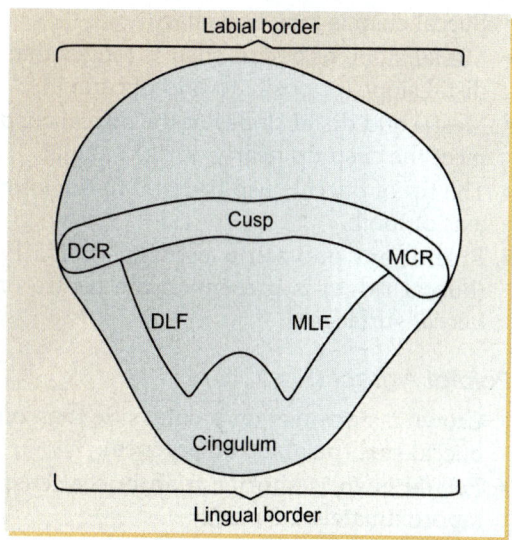

Fig. 1.3e: *Incisal aspect*
MCR: mesial cusp ridge; DCR: distal cusp ridge; MLF: mesial lingual fossa; DLF: distal lingual fossa

- Cusp tip and cusp slopes lie labial to the long axis of the root.

4. First Premolar

Buccal Aspect (Fig. 1.4a)

- Crown is roughly trapezoidal with convex buccal surface.

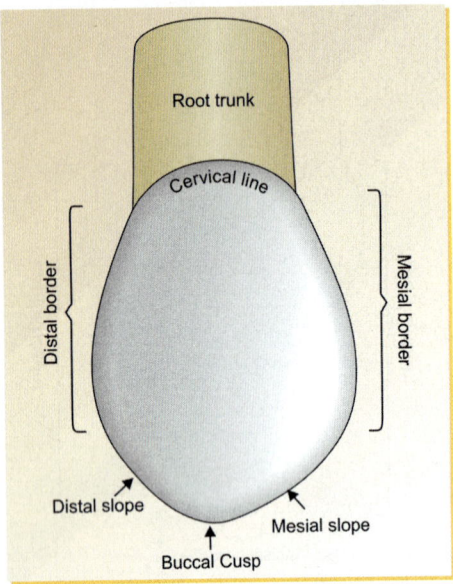

Fig. 1.4a: *Buccal aspect*

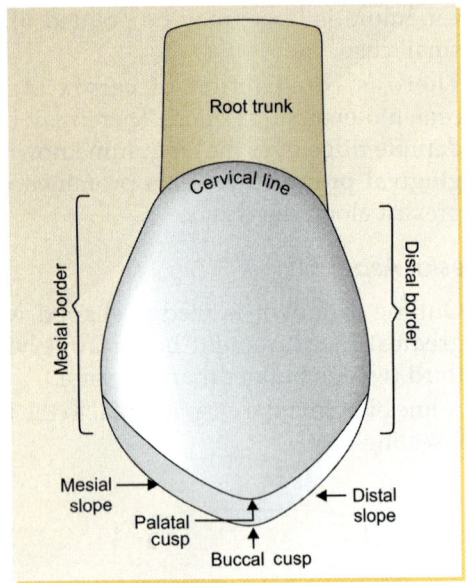

Fig. 1.4b: *Palatal aspect*

- Buccal cusp is long and sharp.
- Mesial slope of buccal cusp is longer than distal slope (opposite to that of canine).
- Mesial and distal slopes of the buccal cusp meet the cusp tip nearly at right angle.
- The tip of buccal cusp is distal to the long axis of tooth.
- Prominent elevation cervico-incisally (buccal ridge) is present in the centre of buccal surface.

Palatal Aspect (Fig. 1.4b)

- Crown is narrower on palatal side than on buccal side (palatal convergence).
- Palatal cusp is shorter than buccal cusp (approximately 1.0 mm).
- Mesial and distal slopes of palatal cusp make rounded angle at cusp tip.

Mesial Aspect (Fig. 1.4c)

- Mesial marginal ridge is occlusally positioned than distal marginal ridge.
- The depression on the mesial surface of the crown is continuous with the depression on the mesial surface of root.
- Mesial developmental depression is present.
- A well-defined developmental groove is seen in the enamel of the mesial marginal ridge.

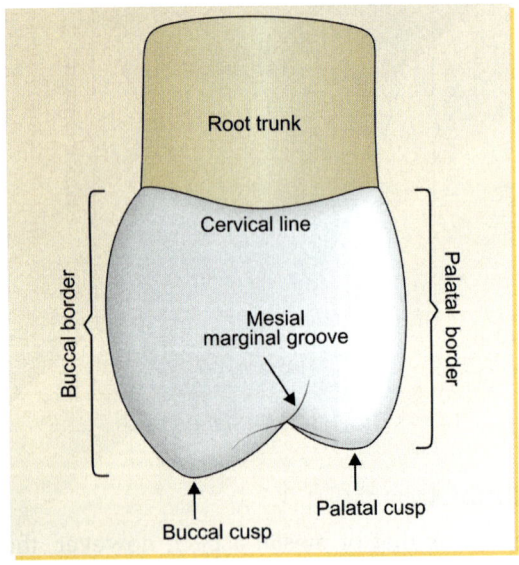

Fig. 1.4c: *Mesial aspect*

Distal Aspect (Fig. 1.4d)

Similar to mesial aspect, with the following differences:

- Distal surface is convex; no depression in the cervical third.
- Cervical line on distal surface has less curvature than the mesial surface.

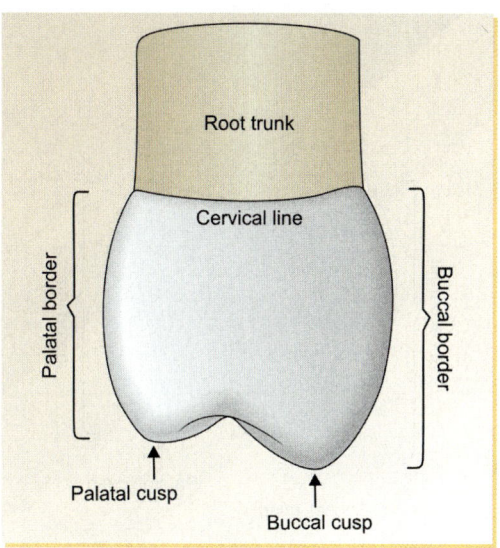

Fig. 1.4d: *Distal aspect*

Occlusal Aspect (Fig. 1.4e)

- Crown is wider on buccal aspect than on the palatal aspect.
- Mesiobuccal cusp ridge joins mesial marginal ridge at almost a right angle and

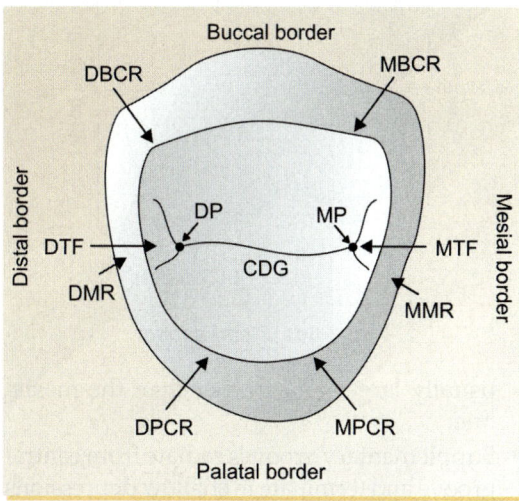

Fig. 1.4e: *Occlusal aspect*

MBCR: mesiobuccal cusp ridge; DBCR: distobuccal cusp ridge; MPCR: mesiopalatal cusp ridge; DPCR: distopalatal cusp ridge; CDG: central developmental groove; MMR: mesial marginal ridge; DMR: distal marginal ridge; MTF: mesial triangular fossa; DTF: distal triangular fossa; MP: mesial pit; DP: distal pit

distobuccal cusp ridge joins distal marginal ridge at acute angle.

- The central groove divides the surface evenly buccolingually. This groove extends from mesial to distal marginal ridge to mesial marginal ridge where it joins mesial marginal groove.
- Distal to mesial marginal ridge, a triangular depression is present known as mesial triangular fossa. The mesiobuccal groove lies in this fossa.
- The triangular depression mesial to distal marginal ridge is called distal triangular fossa. The distobuccal groove lies in this fossa.

Usually the mesial marginal groove crosses mesial marginal ridge (mesial marginal groove connects with the central groove in the mesial triangular fossa).

5. Second Premolar

Buccal Aspect (Fig. 1.5a)

- Crown is about 1.0 mm shorter (less angular and more oblong in shape) than that of first premolar.
- The slopes of buccal cusp are less steep and meet at the cusp tip in a less pointed angle (more obtuse) as compared to first premolar.

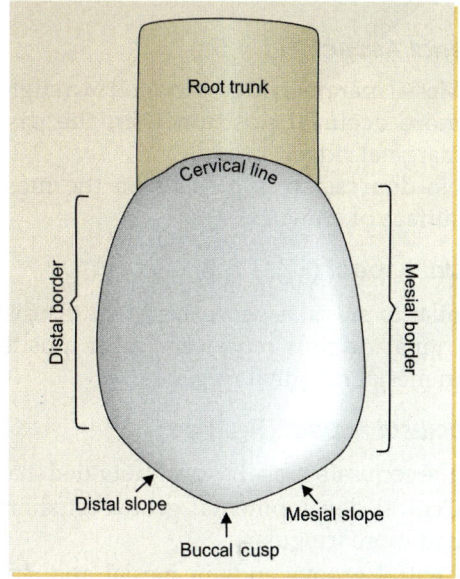

Fig. 1.5a: *Buccal aspect*

- Mesial slope of the buccal cusp is slightly shorter than distal slope (opposite to first premolar and same as that of maxillary canine).

Palatal Aspect (Fig. 1.5b)

- Palatal surface is narrower than buccal surface.
- Palatal and buccal cusp are almost of equal dimensions.

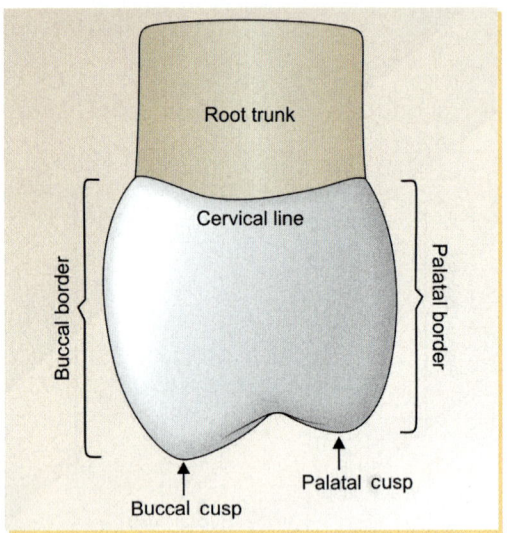

Fig. 1.5c: *Mesial aspect*

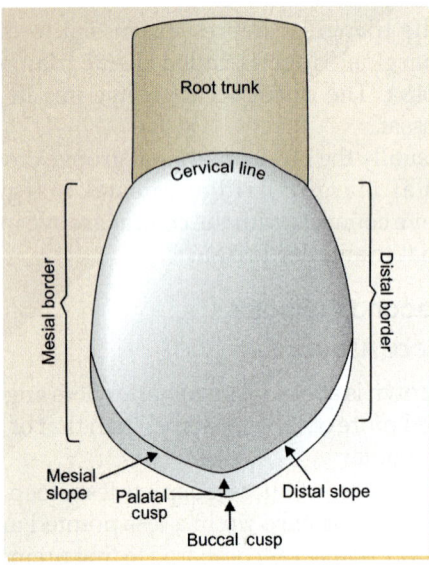

Fig. 1.5b: *Palatal aspect*

Mesial Aspect (Fig. 1.5c)

- Mesial marginal ridge is located in a slightly more occlusal position than the distal marginal ridge.
- No depression is present on the mesial surface of crown.

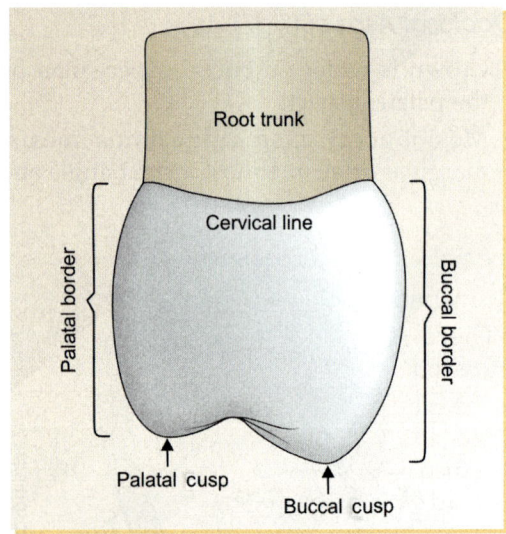

Fig. 1.5d: *Distal aspect*

Distal Aspect (Fig. 1.5d)

Similar to mesial aspect except that the distal marginal ridge is more cervical in position than mesial marginal ridge.

Occlusal Aspect (Fig. 1.5e)

- The occlusal surface has oval/rounded shape.
- Central developmental groove is shorter and more irregular.
- Central groove ends in mesial and distal triangular fossa. Distal triangular fossa is

usually larger and deeper than the mesial one.

- Supplementary grooves radiate from central groove and terminate in shallow depressions (produced wrinkled appearance to the occlusal surface).

6. First Molar

The first molars are the first permanent teeth, which become carious at an early stage and often condemned for extraction.

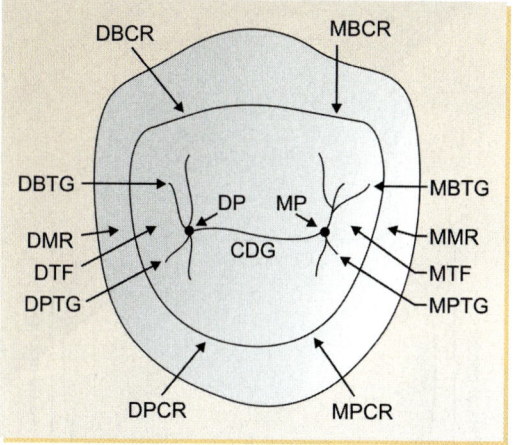

Fig. 1.5e: *Occlusal aspect*
MBCR: mesiobuccal cusp ridge; DBCR: distobuccal cusp ridge; MPCR: mesiopalatal cusp ridge; DPCR: distopalatal cusp ridge; MMR: mesial marginal ridge; DMR: distal marginal ridge; CDG: central developmental groove; MP: mesial pit; DP: distal pit; MTF: mesial triangular fossa; DTF: distal triangular fossa; MBTG: mesiobuccal triangular groove; DBTG: distobuccal triangular groove; MPTG: mesiopalatal triangular groove; DPTG: distopalatal triangular groove

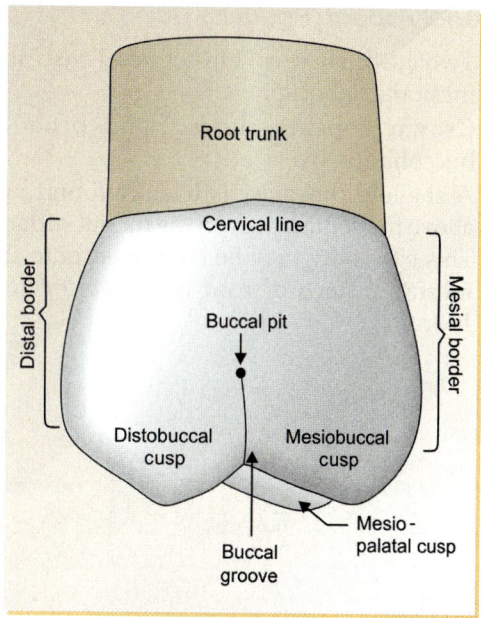

Fig. 1.6a: *Buccal aspect*

Buccal Aspect (Fig. 1.6a)

- Crown is roughly trapezoidal.
- There are two cusps on buccal side: Mesiobuccal and distobuccal.
- The mesiobuccal cusp is broader with the mesial slope meets its distal slope at an obtuse angle. The distobuccal cusp is less broad with the mesial slope meets its distal slope at right angle.
- The parts of mesiopalatal and distopalatal cusps are also visible.
- Buccal groove lies between cusps and extends cervically on the buccal surface to the middle third of crown. At the end of groove is a pit called buccal pit.

Palatal Aspect (Fig. 1.6b)

- Crown is often broader mesiodistally on the palatal surface than on the buccal surface except in the cervical third.
- Two well-defined cusps, mesiopalatal (larger) and distopalatal (smaller) are present.

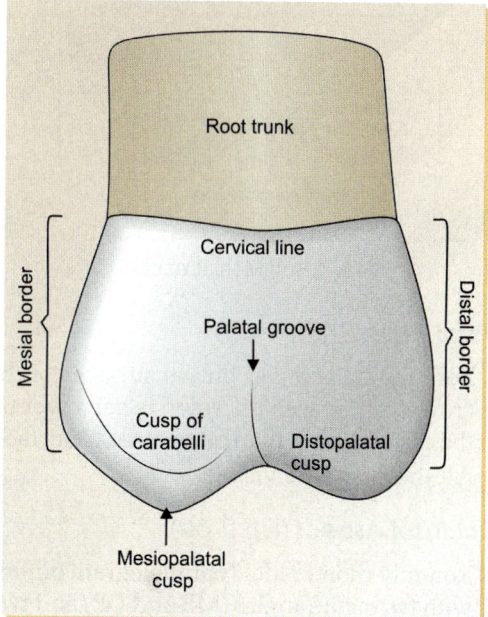

Fig. 1.6b: *Palatal aspect*

- A small cusp may be attached to the palatal surface of mesiopalatal cusp known as **Cusp of Carabelli** or fifth cusp. This fifth cusp is usually 2.0 mm cervical to the tip of mesiopalatal cusp; seen in 60% cases.

Mesial Aspect (Fig. 1.6c)

- Two cusps are seen: Mesiobuccal cusp and mesiopalatal cusp.
- Crown appears shorter and broader buccolingually.
- A shallow concavity is usually found just above the contact area on the mesial surface. This concavity may be continued onto the mesial surface of root trunk at cervical 1/3rd.

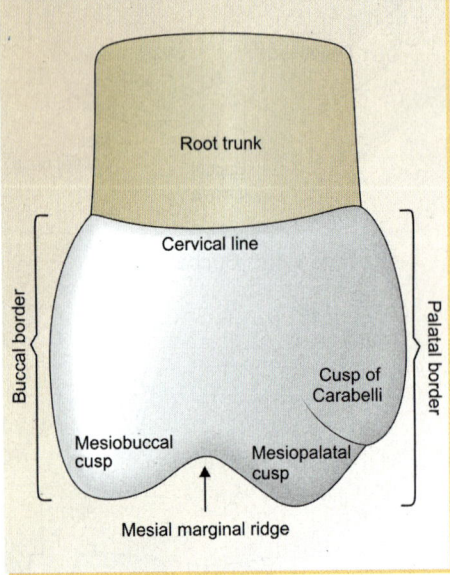

Fig. 1.6c: Mesial aspect

Distal Aspect (Fig. 1.6d)

- Both the palatal and buccal surfaces of the crown can be seen as crown is narrower on the distal surface than on the mesial surface.
- All the cusps are visible.

Occlusal Aspect (Fig. 1.6e)

- Roughly rhomboidal/parallelogram outline with two acute angles (MB and DP) and two obtuse angles (DB and MP).
- Distal surface is narrower buccolingually than mesial surface.
- The main cusp has a triangular ridge. The triangular ridges of the mesiopalatal and distobuccal cusp meet together to form an **Oblique Ridge.**

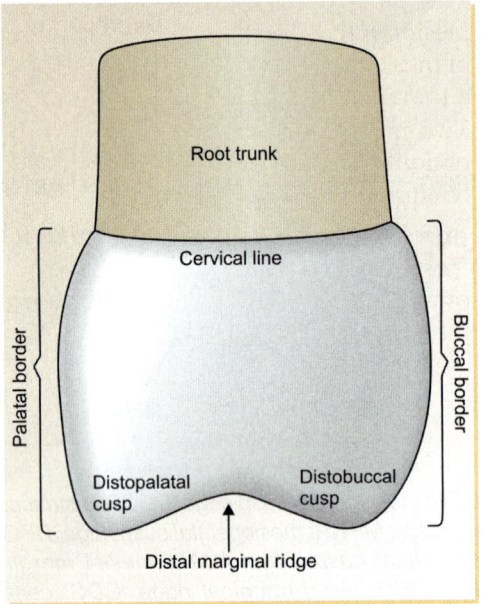

Fig. 1.6d: Distal aspect

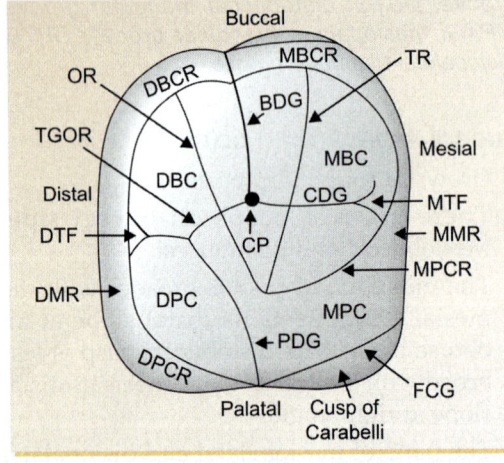

Fig. 1.6e: Occlusal aspect

MBC: mesiobuccal cusp; DBC: distobuccal cusp; MPC: mesiopalatal cusp; DPC: distopalatal cusp; CP: central pit; CDG: central developmental groove; BDG: buccal developmental groove; PDG: palatal developmental groove; FCG: fifth cusp groove; TGOR: transverse groove of oblique ridge; OR: oblique ridge; TR: transverse ridge; MBCR: mesiobuccal cusp ridge; DBCR: distobuccal cusp ridge; MPCR: mesiopalatal cusp ridge; DPCR: distopatalal cusp ridge; MMR: mesial marginal ridge; DMR: distal marginal ridge, MTF: mesial triangular fossa; DTF: distal triangular fossa

- The second triangular ridge of the mesiopalatal cusp and the triangular ridge of mesiobuccal cusp meet together to form a **transverse ridge.**
- Two major fossae; central fossa (mesial to oblique ridge) and distal fossa (distal to oblique ridge).
- Two minor fossae; mesial triangular fossa and distal triangular fossa.
- Four grooves are present; central groove, buccal groove, transverse groove and distal oblique groove.

7. Second Molar

Buccal Aspect (Fig. 1.7a)

- The second molar is slightly smaller than the first molar.
- Mesiobuccal cusp is larger and longer than distobuccal cusp.
- Crown is tilted distally at the cervix. The occlusal surface slants cervically from mesial to distal.
- Buccal groove separates the two buccal cusps, mesiobuccal and distobuccal.

Palatal Aspect (Fig. 1.7b)

- The cusp of Carabelli is absent.

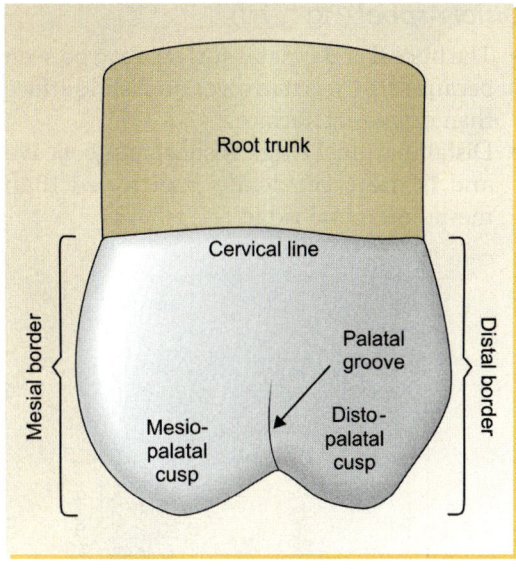

Fig. 1.7b: *Palatal aspect*

- Compared to maxillary first molar, the distopalatal cusp is smaller and the distobuccal cusp may be seen through sulcus between mesiolingual cusp and distolingual cusp.
- Mesiopalatal and distopalatal cusps are visible.

Mesial Aspect (Fig. 1.7c)

- Mesial marginal ridge is longer bucco-palatally and more occlusally located than distal marginal ridge.

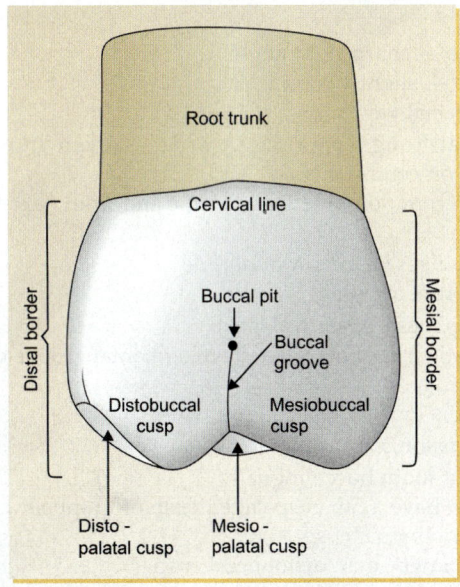

Fig. 1.7a: *Buccal aspect*

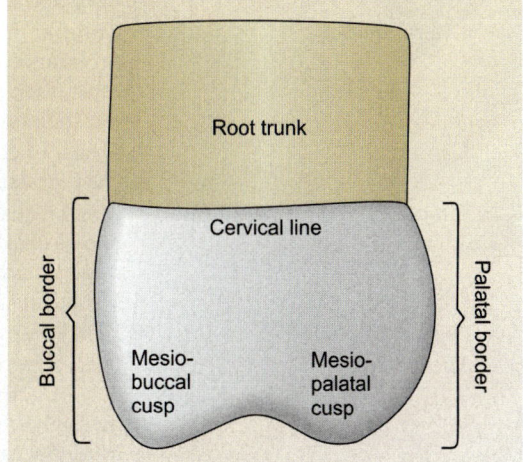

Fig. 1.7c: *Mesial aspect*

Distal Aspect (Fig. 1.7d)

- The buccal and palatal surfaces can be seen because crown is narrower on distal surface than on mesial surface.
- Distal marginal ridge is short and concave and is more cervically positioned than mesial marginal ridge.

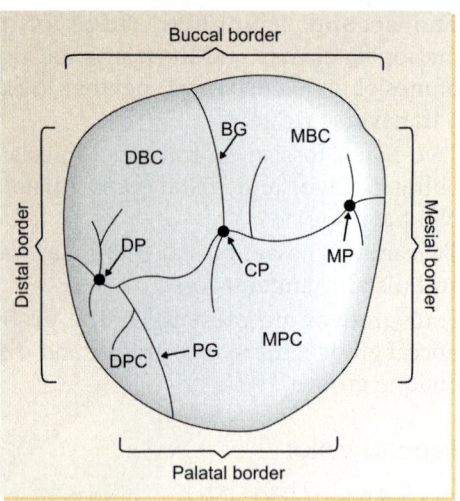

Fig. 1.7e: Occlusal aspect

MBC: mesiobuccal cusp; DBC: distobuccal cusp; MPC: mesiopalatal cusp; DPC: disto palatal cusp; BG: buccal groove; PG: palatal groove; CP: central pit; MP: mesial pit; DP: distal pit

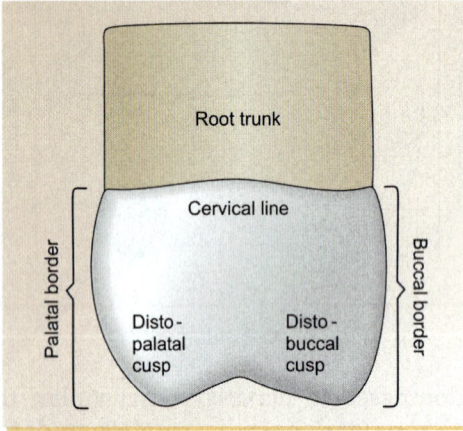

Fig. 1.7d: *Distal aspect*

Occlusal Aspect (Fig. 1.7e)

Occlusally the second molar is similar to the first, except

- Crown is narrower on the palatal side than on the buccal side.
- Crown is narrower on distal side than on the mesial side.
- Fifth cusp is missing.

Maxillary teeth	
Tooth	*Salient features*
Central incisor	• Mesioincisal angle — sharp right angle • Distoincisal angle — slightly round. • Pulp horns — 3 (facial view)
Lateral incisor	• Lingual fossa, although smaller in area, is even more pronounced than on central incisor • Most often shows variation in size and shape and from next to 3rd molars
Canine	• Mesial of crown bulges beyond root outline • Cusp tip labial to root axis line
First premolar	• Lingual cusp tip is mesial to buccal cusp • Shows characteristic mesial marginal developmental groove of mesial marginal ridge • Mesial cusp ridge is longest
Second premolar	• Distal cusp ridge is longest
First molar	• Largest permanent tooth buccolingually • 60% of population have a 5th cusp called cusp of Carabelli on mesial half of mesiolingual cusp • Mesiobuccal cusp larger than distobuccal cusp
Second molar	• Mesiobuccal cusp larger than distobuccal cusp

Differences between maxillary central incisor and maxillary lateral incisor

Maxillary central incisor	Maxillary lateral incisor
Crown:	
• Larger crown	• Smaller crown
• More symmetrical	• Less symmetrical
• Wider mesiodistally	• Mesiodistal and buccolingual dimensions almost same
Mesioincisal angle:	
• Acute (sharp)	• Rounded
Distoincisal angle:	
• Slightly rounded	• More rounded
Lingual fossa:	
• Large but shallow	• Small and deep
Lingual pit:	
• Less frequent	• Commonly seen
Marginal ridges and cingulum	
• Moderately prominent	• More prominent

Difference between maxillary canine and mandibular canine

Maxillary canine	Mandibular canine
• Crown is larger (labiolingual diameter near cervix is greater)	• Crown is less bulky but height is longer
• Mesial and distal margins converge cervically when viewed from labial surface	• Mesial and distal margins are more or less parallel when viewed from labial surface
• Mesial and distal marginal ridges are more accentuated. Lingual ridge and cingulum are prominent.	• Marginal ridges and cingulum are prominent
• Lingual (palatal) fossa is deeper	• Lingual surface is relatively flatter.
• When viewed from mesial or distal aspect, cusp tip lies labial to line passing through cusp tip and root apex	• Cusp tip lies palatal to the line passing through cups tip and long axis of root

Differences between maxillary first and second premolar

First premolar	Second premolar
• Occlusal crown outline is hexagonal	• Occlusal crown outline is ovoid/rounded
• Mesial and distal surfaces converge palatally	• Mesial and distal sides are parallel
• Buccal cusp is higher and bulkier than palatal cusp	• Both cusps are almost equal in height. Palatal cusp is bulkier
• Mesial slope of buccal cusp is longer	• Mesial slope of buccal cusp is shorter
• Mesial and distal pits are placed wider apart. Central groove is longer	• Mesial and distal pits are closer. Central groove is shorter
• Mesial marginal developmental groove interrupts mesial marginal ridge	• There is no mesial marginal developmental groove

How to differentiate between right and left maxillary central incisor
- Mesial profile is straight
- Distal profile is rounded
- Mesioincisal angle is sharp and is nearly a right angle.
- Distoincisal angle is slightly rounded and is obtuse.

Differences between maxillary first and second molar	
First molar	*Second molar*
• Crown is broader on palatal side	• Crown is narrower on palatal side
• Buccal cusps are equal in height	• Distobuccal cusp is smaller
• Distopalatal cusp is large	• Distopalatal cusp is smaller
• Cusp of Carabelli may be present	• Carabelli's cusp is absent
• Occlusal outline is square or rhomboid	• Occlusal outline is rhomboid
• Oblique ridge is prominent	• Oblique ridge is smaller

• Cervical line curves towards incisal surface more on the mesial surface than on distal surface.

How to differentiate between right and left maxillary lateral incisor

• Mesial profile is less rounded
• Distal profile is more rounded
• Distoincisal angle is more rounded than mesioincisal angle

How to differentiate between maxillary right and left canine

• Mesial cusp ridge (mesial slope) is shorter than distal cusp ridge (distal slope)
• Distal surface in entirely convex
• Curvature of cervical line is greater on the mesial surface than on the distal surface.

How to differentiate between right and left maxillary first premolar

• Mesial slope of buccal cusp is straight and longer than distal slope which is shorter and more curved.
• Mesial developmental depression is present.
• A well-defined developmental groove in the enamel of mesial marginal ridge.

How to differentiate between right and left maxillary second premolar

• Mesial slope of buccal cusp is shorter than distal slope (reverse of first premolar).

How to differentiate between right and left maxillary first molar

• The mesiopalatal cusp is largest of all.
• Cusp of Carabelli is present on the palatal surface of mesiopalatal cusp.

• Oblique ridge is present which extends from mesiopalatal cusp to distobuccal cusp.

How to differentiate between right and left maxillary second molar

• Occlusal surface slants cervically from mesial to distal.
• Mesiopalatal cusp is considerably larger in first molar.

MANDIBULAR TEETH

1. Central Incisor

The central incisor is the smallest tooth in dental arch and is bilaterally symmetrical.

Labial Aspect (Fig.1.8a)

• Surface is convex mesiodistally; however flat in incisal third.

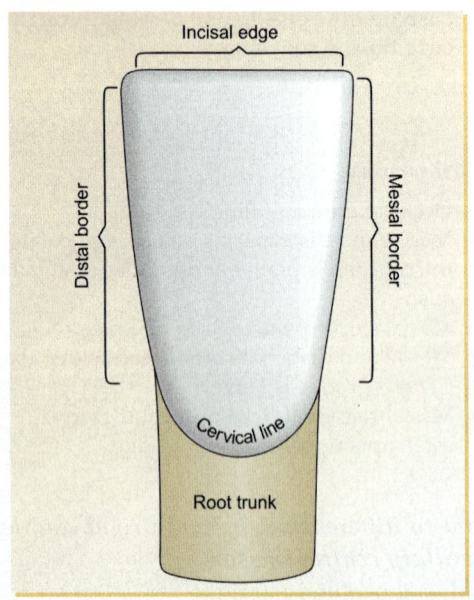

Fig. 1.8a: *Labial aspect*

- Sharp mesial and distal incisal angles.
- Incisal edge of crown is straight and is approximately at right angle to long axis of tooth

Lingual Aspect (Fig.1.8b)

- Crown is narrower lingually (lingual convergence).
- Smooth and slightly concave in the middle and incisal third.
- Cingulum is convex and small.

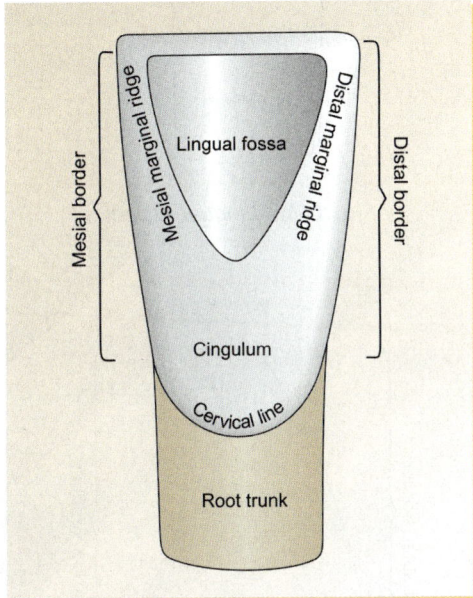

Fig. 1.8b: *Lingual aspect*

Mesial Aspect (Fig.1.8c)

- Crown resembles a wedge. Incisal edge is lingual to the long axis of the root.
- Mesial surface is nearly flat in the cervical and middle thirds, and convex in incisal third.
- Cervical line is deeply curved.

Distal Aspect (Fig.1.8d)

- Shape is similar to that of mesial aspect except that the cervical line curves about 0.5 mm less on distal surface than on mesial surface.

Incisal Aspect (Fig. 1.8e)

- Bilaterally symmetrical.

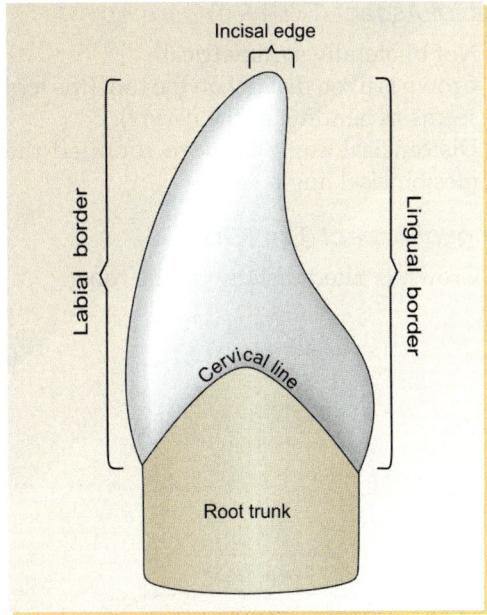

Fig. 1.8c: *Mesial aspect*

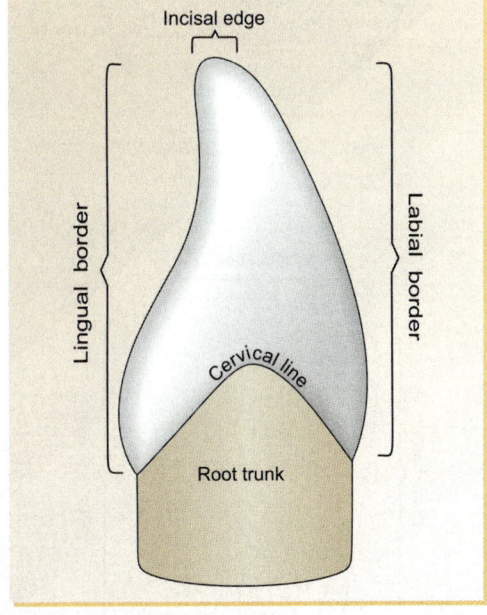

Fig. 1.8d: *Distal aspect*

- Incisal edge is at right angles to the line bisecting the crown labiolingually.

2. Lateral Incisor

Slightly longer than the mandibular central incisor.

Labial Aspect (Fig. 1.9a)

- Not bilaterally symmetrical.
- Crown is tilted distally on the root (the tooth seems as bending at the cervix).
- Distoincisal angle is more rounded than mesioincisal angle.

Lingual Aspect (Fig. 1.9b)

- Crown is tilted distally on the root.

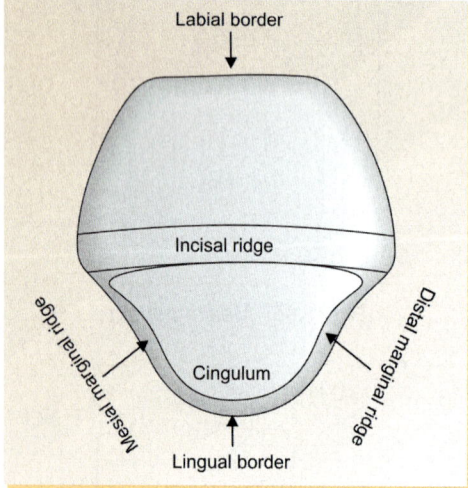

Fig. 1.8e: *Incisal aspect*

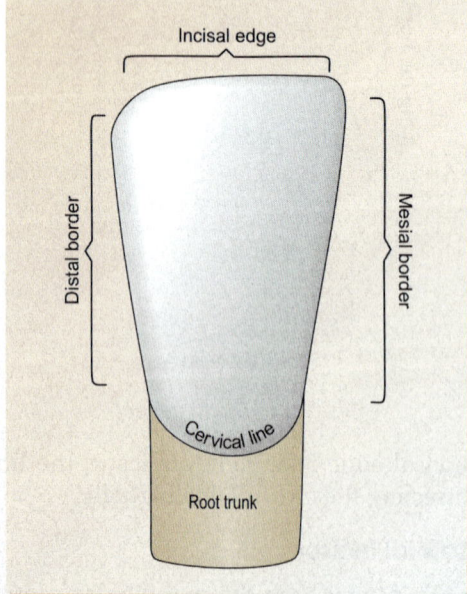

Fig. 1.9a: *Labial aspect*

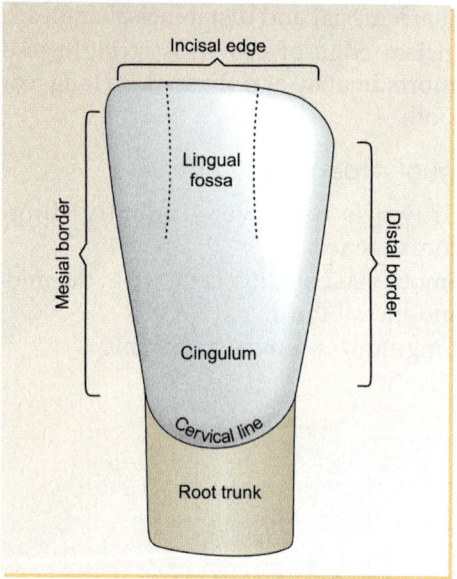

Fig. 1.9b: *Lingual aspect*

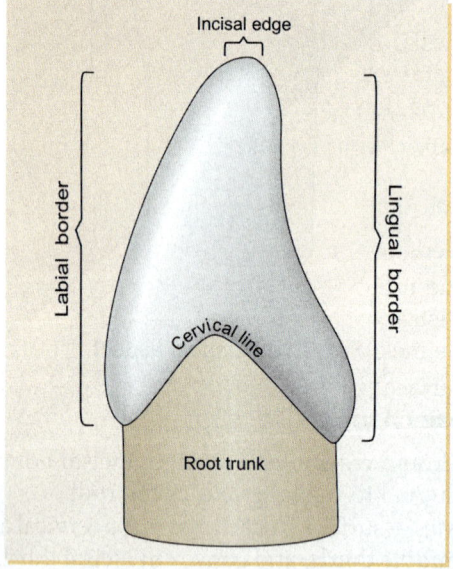

Fig. 1.9c: *Mesial aspect*

- Mesial marginal ridge is slightly larger than the distal marginal ridge.
- Cingulum lies distal to the long axis of tooth.

Mesial Aspect (Fig. 1.9c)

- Wedge shaped
- Incisal edge is slightly lingual to the long axis of the root.

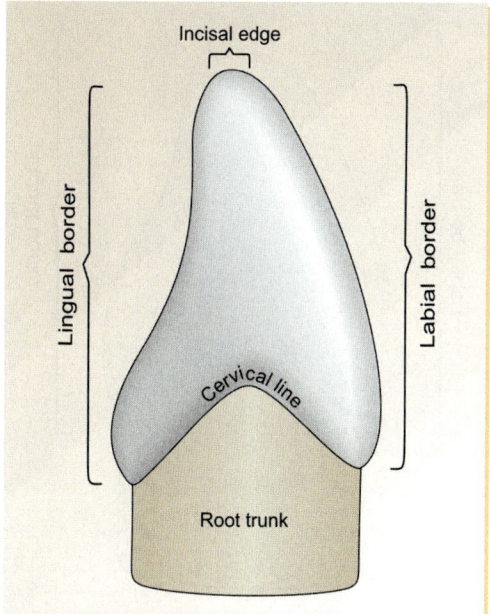

Fig. 1.9d: *Distal aspect*

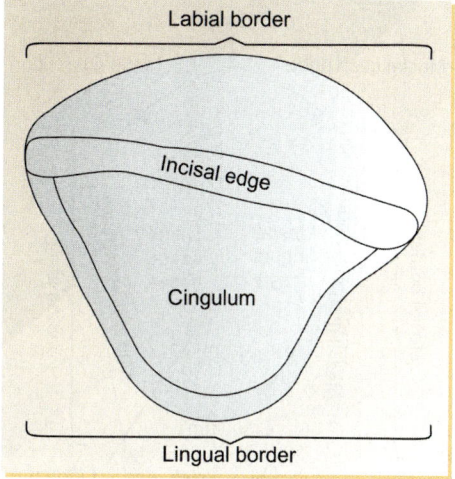

Fig. 1.9e: *Incisal aspect*

- Mesial side of crown in often longer than distal side which causes incisal edge to slope downward in a distal direction.
- Cervical line curvature is deep.

Distal Aspect (Fig. 1.9d)

- Wedge shaped.
- The incisal edge is twisted distolingually (distal portion is more lingually placed than the mesial portion).
- Cervical line curvature 0.5 mm less deep than on mesial surface.

Incisal Aspect (Fig.1.9e)

- Not bilaterally symmetrical.
- The incisal edge has distolingual twist (distal end of incisal edge is bent lingually). This twist of incisal edge corresponds to the curvature of mandibular dental arch.

3. Canine

Canines are larger than the incisors.

Labial Aspect (Fig. 1.10a)

- Crown appears long and narrow (compared with maxillary canine).

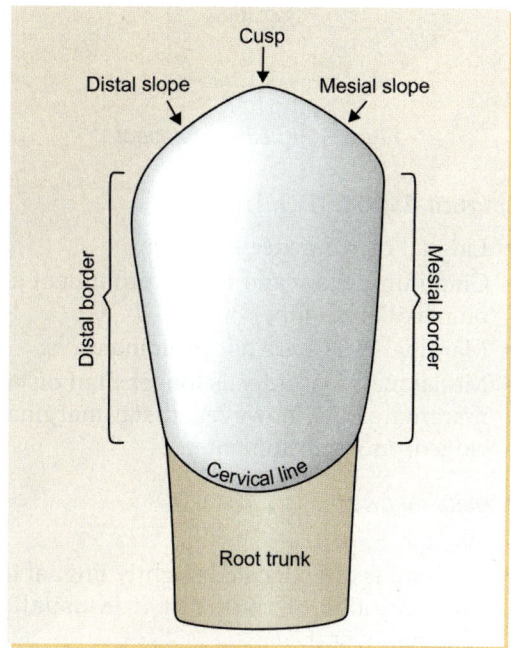

Fig. 1.10a: *Labial aspect*

- Labial surface is convex. A labial ridge, less pronounced than maxillary canine, is present.
- There is more of crown distal to the long axis of root than mesial to it (crown appears to be tilted distally).
- Mesial slope of the cusp is shorter than distal slope (same as that of maxillary canine).

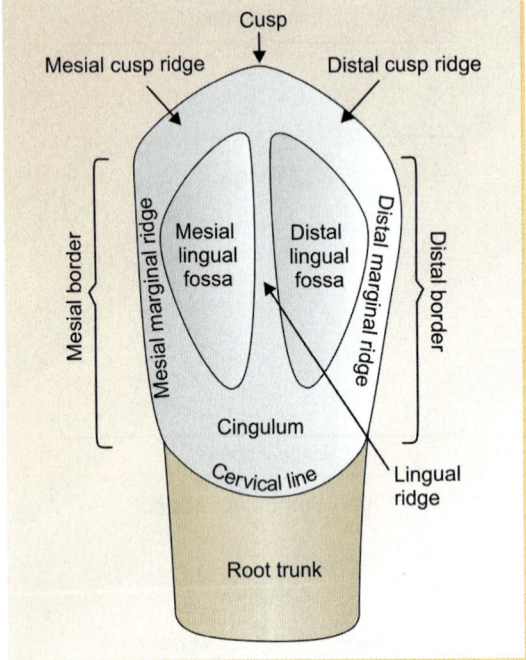

Fig. 1.10b: *Lingual aspect*

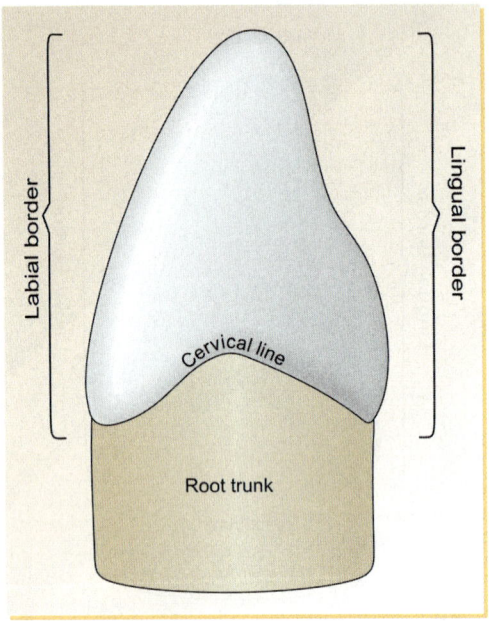

Fig. 1.10c: *Mesial aspect*

Lingual Aspect (Fig. 1.10b)

- Lingual convergence is present.
- Cingulum is low and not as prominent as on maxillary canines.
- Marginal ridges are not prominent.
- Mesial marginal ridge is longer than distal marginal ridge; however, distal marginal ridge is more prominent.

Mesial Aspect (Fig.1.10c)

- Wedge-shaped
- Cusp tip is often located slightly lingual to the long axis of root, but it is usually centered over it.
- Cervical line curvature is more than on maxillary canines.

Distal Aspect (Fig.1.10d)

Similar to the mesial aspect except that the:
- Cervical line has about 1.0 mm less curvature on the distal surface than on the mesial surface.
- Distolingual angle is slightly lingual in position than the cusp tip (the crown is twisted distolingually).

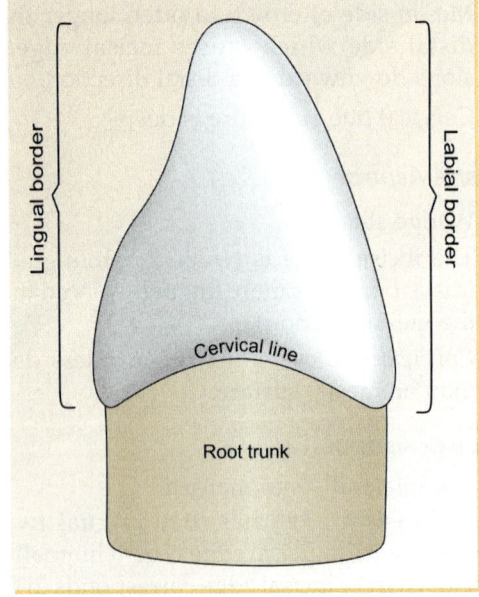

Fig. 1.10d: *Mesial aspect*

Incisal Aspect (Fig.1.10e)

- Cusp tip is near the centre labiolingually or may be lingual to the centre.
- Distoincisal angle is lingually placed and the tooth appears to be twisted disolingually.

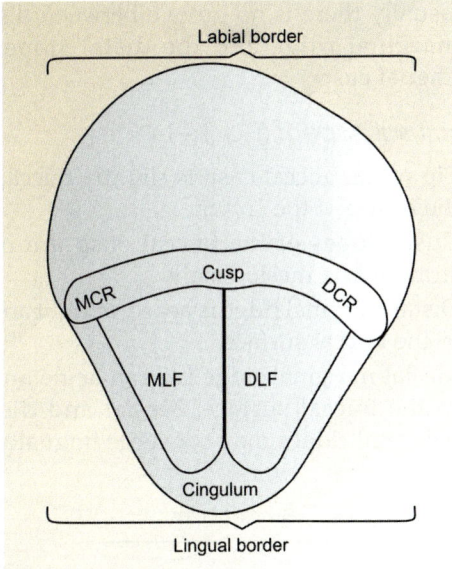

Fig. 1.10e: *Incisal aspect*

MCR: mesial cusp ridge; DCR: distal cusp ridge; MLF: mesial lingual fossa; DLF: distal lingual fossa

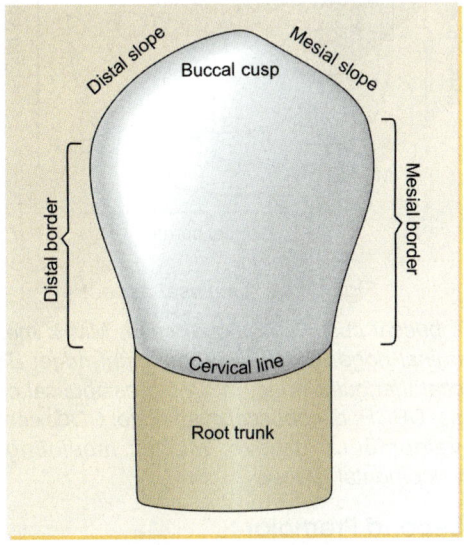

Fig. 1.11a: *Buccal aspect*

4. First Premolar

Buccal Aspect (Fig. 1.11a)

- Appears symmetrical except for the distal tilt of the crown.
- Buccal cusp tip is located near the long axis of tooth with mesial cusp slope slightly shorter than distal cusp slope.

- Buccal cusp is long and sharp, the cusp slopes meet at an obtuse angle.

Lingual Aspect (Fig. 1.11b)

- Lingual convergence is prominent.
- Lingual cusp is small and pointed.
- Mesial marginal ridge is more cervically located than distal marginal ridge (only tooth with this characteristic).
- The mesiolingual groove separates the mesial marginal ridge from the mesial slope of the lingual cusp.

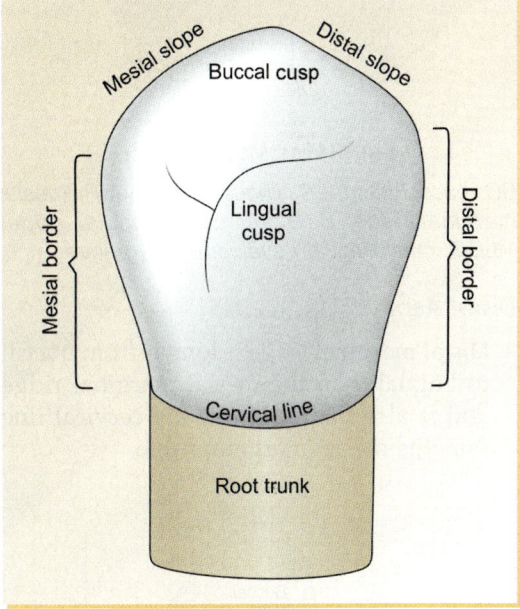

Fig. 1.11b: *Lingual aspect*

Mesial Aspect (Fig.1.11c)

- Crown is tilted lingually.
- Tip of the buccal cusp is often centered over the long axis of the root.
- Triangular ridge of the buccal cusp slopes cervically at 45 degree angle from the cusp tip towards the centre of the occlusal surface.
- Mesiolingual groove is present between the mesial marginal ridge and mesial slope of lingual cusp.
- Mesial marginal ridge is usually located more cervically than distal marginal ridge.

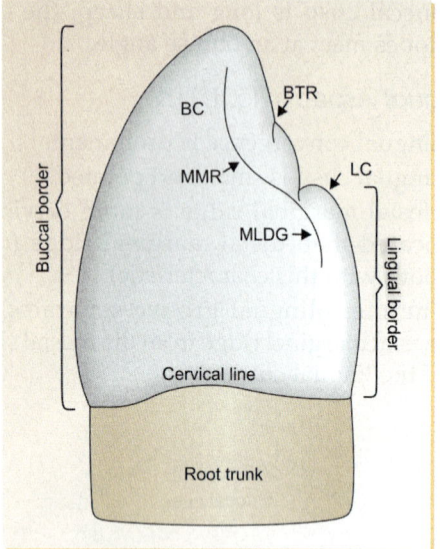

Fig. 1.11c: *Mesial aspect*

BC: buccal cusp; LC: lingual cusp; MMR: mesial marginal ridge; BTR: buccal triangular ridge; MLDG: mesiolingual developmental groove

Distal Aspect (Fig. 1.11d)

- Distal marginal ridge is longer from buccal to lingual than the mesial marginal ridge and is also placed above the cervical line than the mesial marginal ridge.

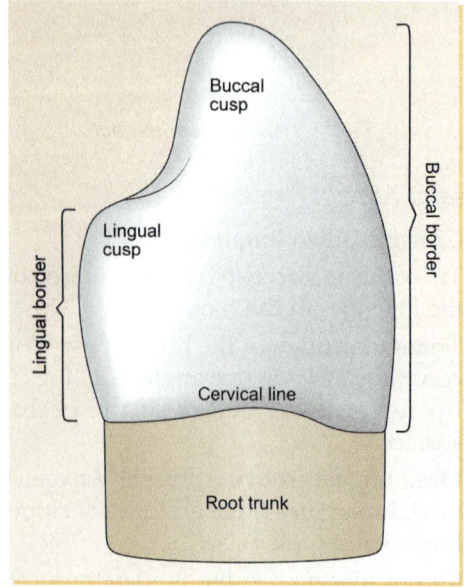

Fig. 1.11d: *Distal aspect*

- Usually there is no groove between distal marginal ridge and the distal slope of lingual cusp.

Occlusal Aspect (Fig. 1.11e)

- Tip of the buccal cusp is slightly buccal to the centre of the crown.
- Cusp slopes of the buccal cusp are in a straight line mesiodistally.
- Distal marginal ridge is nearly at right angle to the buccal surface.
- Mesial marginal ridge is at an acute angle to the buccal surface. Mesial and distal marginal ridges may converge lingually.

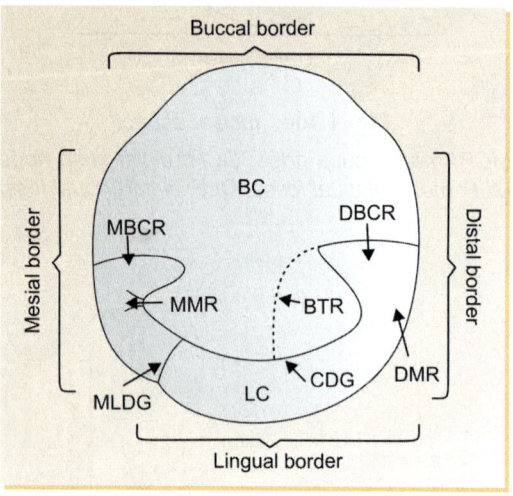

Fig. 1.11e: *Occlusal aspect*

BC: buccal cusp; LC: lingual cusp; MMR: mesial marginal ridge; DMR: distal marginal ridge; BTR: buccal triangular ridge; MBCR: mesiobuccal cusp ridge; DBCR: distobuccal cusp ridge; CDG: central developmental groove; MLDG: mesiolingual developmental groove

5. Second Premolar

Two types of second premolars; two cusp type or three cusp type are prevalent.

Buccal Aspect (Fig. 1.12a)

- Almost squarish in appearance. Surface is convex with inconspicuous buccal ridge.
- Buccal cusp is less pointed as compared to the mandibular first premolar and the cusp slopes are less steep.

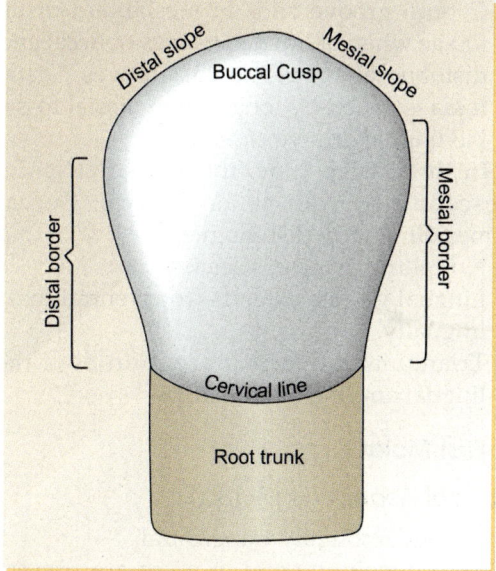

Fig. 1.12a: *Buccal aspect*

- Contact area is occlusally located as compared to first premolar.

Lingual Aspect (Fig. 1.12b)

A. One buccal and one lingual cusp
  - Lingual cusp is smaller than buccal cusp; however, larger than that of first premolar.

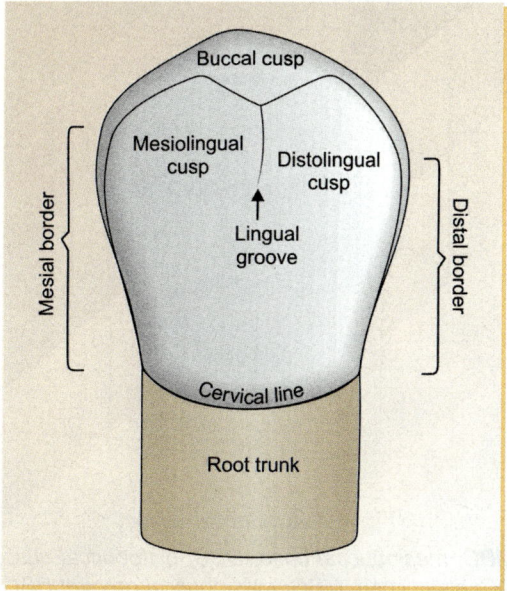

Fig. 1.12b: *Lingual aspect*

- Lingual cusp is either mesial to or along the long axis of the root.
- Distal marginal ridge is cervically located than mesial marginal ridge.

B. One buccal cusp and two lingual cusps
  - Lingual configuration may be same as that of buccal or even wider.
  - Mesiolingual cusp is longer than distolingual cusp.
  - Groove is present between mesiolingual and distolingual cusps.

Mesial Aspect (Fig.1.12c)

As compared to first premolar
- Crown and root are wider buccolingually.
- Buccal cusp is not so nearly centered over root.
- Lingual lobe development is greater.
- No mesiolingual developmental groove.

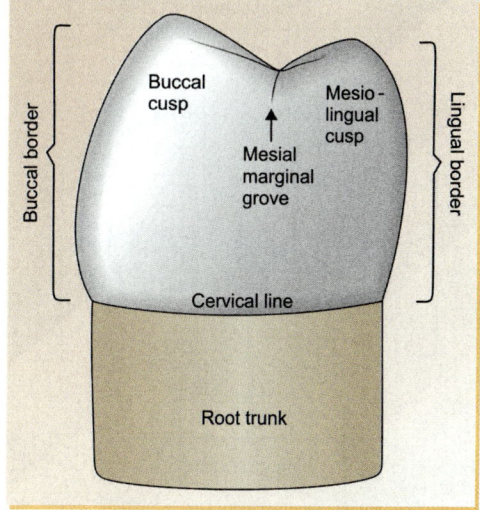

Fig. 1.12c: *Mesial aspect*

Distal Aspect (Fig.1.12d)

Resembles mesial aspect except
- Cervical line is 0.2 mm less curved on distal surface than on mesial surface.
- In three cusp tooth, the distolingual cusp is smaller than the mesiolingual cusp.

Occlusal Aspect (Fig.1.12e)

In two cusp type
- Lingual cusp is smaller than buccal cusp.

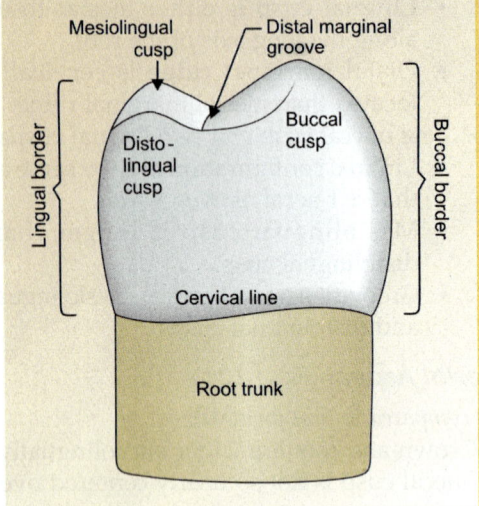

Fig. 1.12d: *Distal aspect*

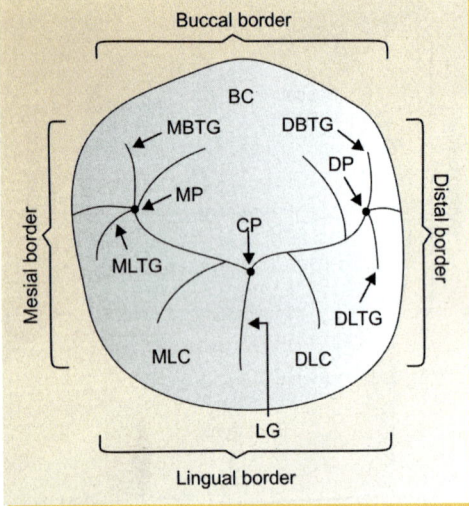

Fig. 1.12e: *Occlusal aspect*

BC: buccal cusp; MLC: mesiolingual cusp; DLC: distolingual cusp; MBTG: mesiobuccal triangular groove; DBTG: distobuccal triangular groove; MLTG: mesiolingual triangular groove; DLTG: distolingual triangular groove; LG: lingual groove; CP: central pit; MP: mesial pit; DP: distal pit

- Central groove extends mesiodistally across the occlusal surface.
- The triangular ridge is large on the buccal cusp than on lingual cusp.
- No central fossa is seen.

- Central groove ends in mesial and distal fossae where it often joins mesiobuccal and distobuccal supplemental grooves. Distal fossa is generally longer than mesial fossa.
- No lingual groove is seen.

  In three cusp type, the size of cusps in descending order is as follows: Buccal > mesiolingual > distolingual
- No central groove is seen.
- Lingual groove extends from central fossa lingually.
- Triangular ridge is present on both the lingual and the buccal cusps.

6. First Molar

Buccal Aspect (Fig.1.13a)

- Crown is roughly trapezoidal.
- Two developmental grooves are present viz. mesiobuccal developmental groove and distobuccal developmental groove. Mesiobuccal developmental groove acts as line of demarcation between mesiobuccal lobe and distobuccal lobe. Distobuccal developmental groove separates distobuccal lobe from distal lobe.
- Buccal cusps are usually flattened.

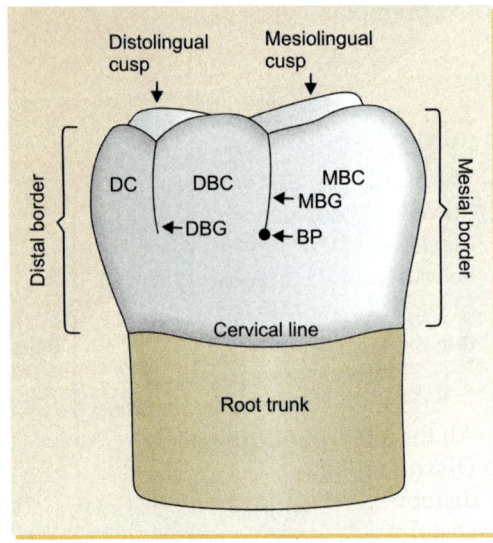

Fig. 1.13a: *Buccal aspect*

MBC: mesiobuccal cusp; DBC: distobuccal cusp; DC: distal cusp; MBG: mesiobuccal groove; DBG: Distobuccal groove; BP: buccal pit

Lingual Aspect (Fig.1.13b)

- Crown tapers towards lingual side (lingual convergence).
- From lingual aspect, three cusps may be seen, two lingual cusps and lingual portion of distal cusp.
- Mesiolingual cusp is widest mesiodistally with its cusp tip placed at higher level than distolingual cusp.
- Lingual groove separates mesiolingual cusp from distolingual cusp.

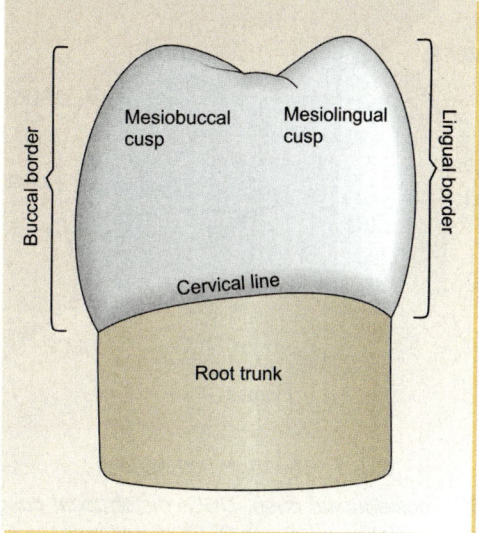

Fig. 1.13c: *Mesial aspect*

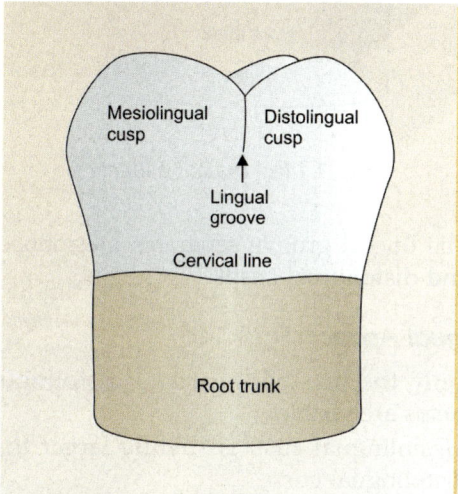

Fig. 1.13b: *Lingual aspect*

Mesial Aspect (Fig.1.13c)

- Two cusps are seen.
- Lingual tilt is evident
- The buccal surface has a bulge in the cervical third, known as buccal cervical ridge.
- Mesial marginal ridge is concave and may be crossed by a groove.
- Mesiolingual cusp is sharp as compared to mesiobuccal cusp.

Distal Aspect (Fig. 1.13d)

- All the cusps can be seen.
- Distolingual cusp is longer than the distobuccal cusp.
- Distal marginal ridge is short and located lingual and distal to the distal cusp. It is cervically located than mesial marginal ridge.
- The distal cusp, which is on the distobuccal angle of the crown is smallest of the five cusps.

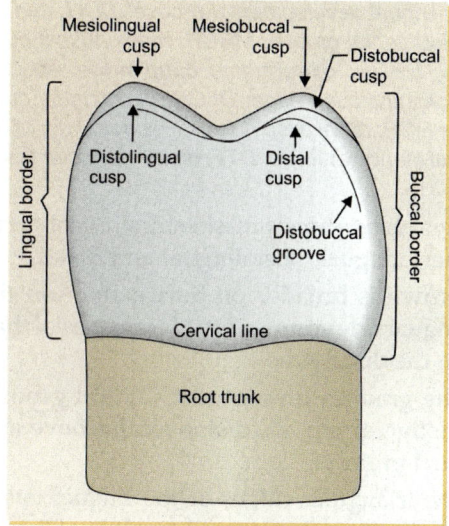

Fig. 1.13d: *Distal aspect*

- Mesiolingual cusp (usually the largest) is visible behind the mesiobuccal cusp.
- Distolingual cusp is visible behind the distobuccal cusp.
- Occlusal surface slopes cervically from mesial to distal (distally tipping).

Occlusal Aspect (Fig.1.13e)

- Somewhat hexagonal in shape.
- It is always larger in dimension mesiodistally than buccolingually.

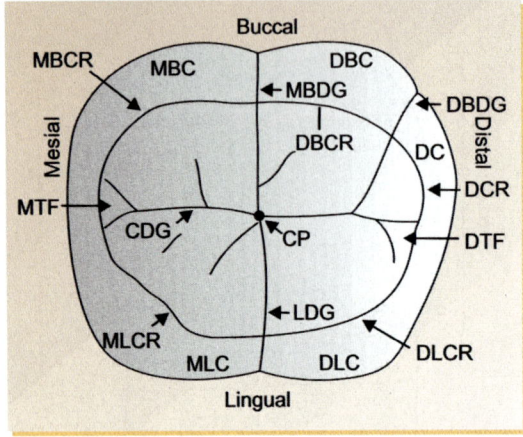

Fig. 1.13e: *Occlusal aspect*

MBC: mesiobuccal cusp; DBC: distobuccal cusp; MLC: mesiolingual cusp; DLC: distolingual cusp; DC: distal cusp; MBDG: mesiobuccal developmental groove; DBDG: distobuccal developmental groove LDG: lingual developmental groove; CDG: central developmental groove; MBCR: mesiobuccal cusp ridge; DBCR: distobuccal cusp ridge; MLCR: mesiolingual cusp ridge; DLCR: distolingual cusp ridge; DCR: distal cusp ridge; CP: central pit; MTF: mesial triangular fossa; DTF: distal triangular fossa

- Five cusps, namely mesiobuccal, distobuccal, mesiolingual, distolingual and distal.
- Crown is broader on buccal than on the lingual side and also broader on mesial than on the distal side.

  The grooves present are: Central groove, mesiobuccal groove, distobuccal groove and lingual groove

  The triangular ridges of the lingual cusps are longer than the triangular ridges of buccal cusps and triangular ridges of mesiobuccal cusp and mesiolingual cusp join to form a transverse ridge.

7. Second Molar

Buccal Aspect (Fig. 1.14a)

Crown is somewhat shorter cervico-occlusally and narrower mesiodistally than in the first molar.

- All the four cusps viz. mesiobuccal, distobuccal, mesiolingual and distolingual are visible.

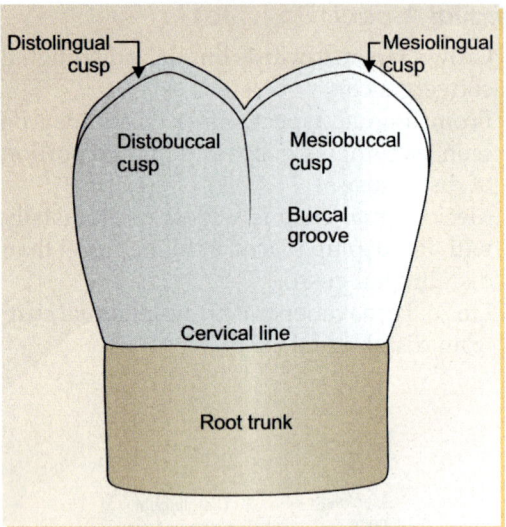

Fig. 1.14a: *Buccal aspect*

- The buccal groove separates mesiobuccal and distobuccal cusps.

Lingual Aspect (Fig.1.14b)

- Only the mesiolingual and distolingual cusps are visible.
- Mesiolingual cusp is slightly larger than distolingual cusp.
- Crown is slightly narrower on lingual side than on the buccal side.

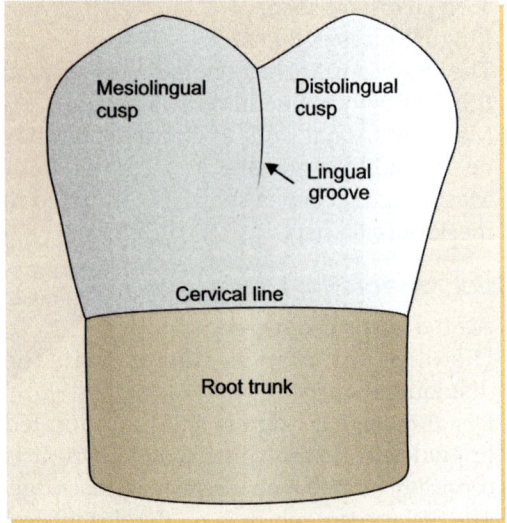

Fig. 1.14b: *Lingual aspect*

Mesial Aspect (Fig.1.14c)

- Mesiolingual cusp is the longest cusp.
- Mesiobuccal cusp is shorter than mesiolingual cusp.
- Mesial marginal ridge is concave and is not crossed by a groove.

Distal Aspect (Fig.1.14d)

- Tips of mesiobuccal and mesiolingual cusps can be seen.
- Distobuccal cusp is shortest of the four cusps.
- The crown tilts distally; the distal marginal ridge is more cervically located.

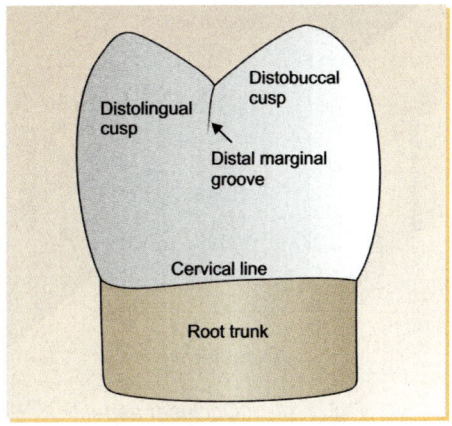

Fig. 1.14d: *Distal aspect*

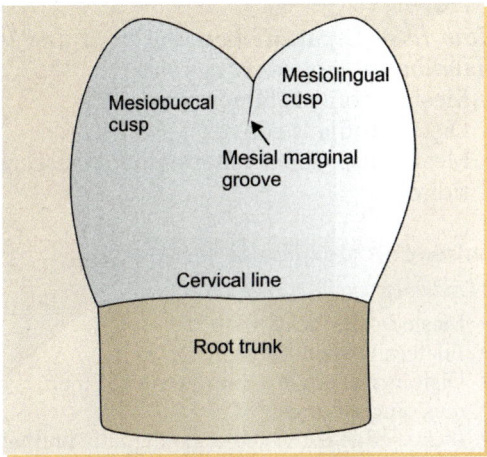

Fig. 1.14c: *Mesial aspect*

Occlusal Aspect (Fig.1.14e)

- The crown has a rectangular shape and is larger mesiodistally than buccolingually.
- Crown tapers both lingually and distally
- The buccal surface of mesiobuccal cusp often has a prominent bulge (mesial cervical ridge).
- The triangular ridges of mesiobuccal and mesiolingual cusps form a transverse ridge and also the triangular ridges of distobuccal and distolingual cusps form a transverse ridge.

The grooves present are: Central groove, buccal groove and lingual groove.

Mandibular teeth	
Tooth	*Salient features*
Central incisor	• Smallest of all teeth
Later incisor	• Incisal edge follows curvature of dental arch giving crown appearance of being twisted slightly on its root base
Canine	• Mesial cusp ridge almost horizontal
First premolar	• Crown has lingual tilt of 30° to long axis of root
	• Shows a characteristic 'mesiolingual developmental groove'
	• Mesial marginal ridge is lower than distal
Second premolar	• Y groove pattern on 3 cusp type
	• H or U groove pattern on 2 cusp type
First molar	• Greatest mesiodistal diameter of all teeth
	• Pentagonal in shape occlusally
Second molar	• Buccal and lingual grooves alight to intersect with central groove like a "+" (plus)

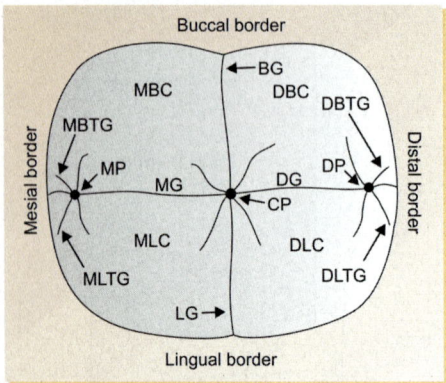

Fig. 1.14e: *Occlusal aspect*

MBC: mesiobuccal cusp; DBC: distobuccal cusp; MLC: mesiolingual cusp; DLC: distolingual cusp; BG: buccal groove; LG: lingual groove; MG: mesial groove; DG: distal groove; MBTG: mesiobuccal triangular groove; MLTG: mesiolingual triangular groove; DBTG: distobuccal triangular groove; DLTG: distolingual triangular groove; CP: central pit; MP: mesial pit; DP: distal pit

How to differentiate between right and left mandibular central incisors
Curvature of cervical line is more on mesial surface than on distal surface.

How to differentiate between right and left mandibular lateral incisors
- Incisal edge slopes downward in distal direction
- Mesial side of crown is often longer than distal side
- A tendency towards deep concavity on distal side of mandibular lateral incisor above cervical line is present.
- Incisal edge is twisted distolingually on the crown

How to differentiate between right and left mandibular permanent canines
- Mesial profile is almost straight
- Distal profile is convex
- Mesial cusp ridge is shorter than distal cusp ridge

Differences between mandibular central incisor and mandibular lateral incisor

Mandibular central incisor	*Mandibular lateral incisor*
• Mesiodistally narrower	• Mesiodistally wider
• Bilaterally symmetrical	• Bilaterally asymmetrical
• Mesioincisal and distoincisal angles are sharp and at right angle	• Distoincisal angle is more rounded than mesioincisal angle
• Incisal edge is at right angle to labiolingual bisecting line	• Incisal edge is twisted distolingually on the crown

Differences between mandibular first and second premolars

First premolar	*Second premolar*
• Occlusal outline is diamond shaped	• Occlusal outline is squarish or triangular
• Mesial and distal margins converge lingually	• Mesial and distal margins are parallel
• Buccal cusp is prominent and lingual cusp is rudimentary	• Both cusps are equal in size
• Central pit is never present	• Central pit may be present (in 3 cusp type)
• Transverse ridge is between buccal and lingual cusps	• No transverse ridge is seen
• Occlusal surface slopes lingually	• Occlusal surface is horizontal
• Mesiolingual developmental groove is present	• Mesiolingual groove is generally absent

Differences between mandibular first and second molars

First molar	*Second molar*
• Occlusal outline pentagonal or hexagonal	• Occlusal outline rectangular
• Generally 5 cusps are present, 3 buccal and 2 lingual	• Four cusps are present. Distal cusp is absent.
• Two buccal grooves are present	• One buccal groove is present
• Main occlusal grooves form a Y-pattern	• Main grooves form a + pattern
• Mesiodistally very wide	• Mesiodistally smaller

How to differentiate between right and left mandibular first premolar
- Mesiolingual groove is present
- Occlusal surface slopes lingually

How to differentiate between right and left mandibular second premolar
Two cusp type
- Occlusal outline is rounded and somewhat oval.
- There is often a depression separating the distal marginal ridge from the lingual cusp.
- Distal marginal ridge is usually more cervical in position than the mesial marginal ridge.
- Distal fossa is generally larger than mesial fossa.
- Cervical line is more curved on mesial surface than on the distal surface

Three cusp type
- Occlusal outline is more square or angular.

- Distolingual cusp is usually smaller than mesiolingual cusp.
- Distal groove is shorter than mesial groove.
- Central fossa is distal to the centre of the occlusal surface.

How to differentiate between right and left mandibular first molar
- Buccal surface has two developmental grooves.
- Lingual surface is comparatively smoother
- A small distal cusp is present on occlusal surface

How to differentiate between right and left mandibular second molar
- Crown tilts distally, causing the occlusal surface to slope cervically from mesial to distal
- Crown tapers both distally as well as lingually.

Contact areas

Maxillary teeth	Mesial	Diagrammatic representation	Distal
Central incisor	In the incisal third, very near the incisal edge.	1 1 2	Near the junction of incisal and middle thirds.
Lateral incisor	In the incisal third	1 2 3	At junction of incisal and middle-third
Canine	At the junction of incisial and middle thirds, closer to cusp tip than distal contact point	2 3 4	In the middle-third just cervical to the junction of incisal and middle thirds. Often it is in the middle of middle third and is more cervically located than the meisal contact point
First premolar	Usually in the middle third at or just cervical to the junction of occlusal and middle third	3 4 5	In the middle third, slightly more cervical in position than mesial contact area
Second premolar	Near the junction of middle and occlusal thirds	4 5 6	Slightly more cervical in position than mesial contact area.
First molar	At the junction of the occlusal and middle third	5 6 7	At the middle of middle third, cervical to mesial one
Second molar	At the junction of occlusal and middle third	6 7 8	At the middle of middle third

(contd.)

Contact areas (contd.)

Mandibular teeth	Mesial	Diagrammatic representation	Distal
Central incisor	In the incisal third, near the mesioincisal angle almost level with the incisal edge	1 1 2	In the incisal third, about the same level as the mesial contact area
Lateral incisor	In the incisal third, fairly near incisal edge	1 2 3	In the incisal third, but cervical to the level of mesial contact area
Canine	In the incisal third just below the mesioincisal angle	2 3 4	At the junction of middle and incisal third more cervically located than the mesial contact area
First premolar	At the junction of occlusal and middle thirds or slightly cervical to it	3 4 5	Distal contact area is usually slightly more occlusal in position than mesial contact area
Second premolar	Occlusal to junction of occlusal and middle third	4 5 6	At the same level or slightly cervical to mesial contact area
First molar	At the junction of the occlusal and middle third	5 6 7	Beneath the distal cusp, near the middle of the middle third
Second molar	About the junction of middle and occlusal third	6 7 8	The centre of the middle third of the total crown length

2

Dental Caries

Nature has provided us teeth to perform the functions of cutting, grinding and admixing food with saliva. The hard enamel cover along with the periodontal ligament can withstand forces of mastication. It is very strange that the hardest tissue of the body — the enamel, which is indestructible otherwise, can disintegrate in the oral environment. *Caries* (Latin meaning 'dry rot') is the name *given to the process of slow disintegration that may affect any of the biological hard tissue as a result of bacterial action.* Rarely this action may affect bone, causing bone caries. Usually such disintegration affects enamel, dentin and cementum — *the tooth* — that is why the term dental caries is most common.

DEFINITIONS

Dental caries is peculiarly a local disease, which involves destruction of hard tissues of the teeth by metabolites produced by oral micro-organisms.

Dental caries can be defined as *the irreversible, slow progressing decay of hard tissues of the tooth.* It can be defined as *the microbial disease of the calcified tissues of teeth, characterized by demineralization of the inorganic portion and destruction of organic substance of the tooth* (Shafer).

According to WHO, caries is defined as *a localized post eruptive, pathological process of external origin involving softening of the hard tooth tissue and proceeding to the formation of a cavity.*

Classification of Caries

Dental caries can be classified according to six major factors:

A. According to morphology of teeth
B. According to severity of lesion
C. According to progress of lesion
D. According to virginity of lesion
E. According to age pattern
F. Based on WHO system

A. According to Morphology of Teeth

a. *Pit and fissure caries*: Caries occurring on anatomical pits and fissures of all the teeth (Figs 2.1 to 2.3).

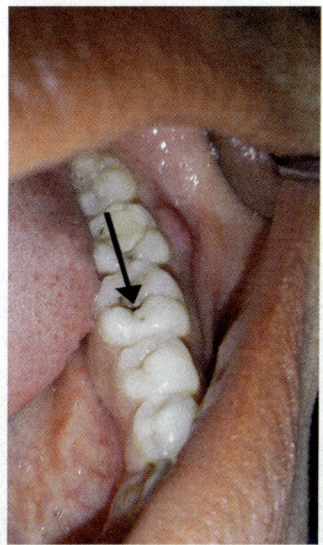

Fig. 2.1: *Pit and fissure caries involving occlusal surface*

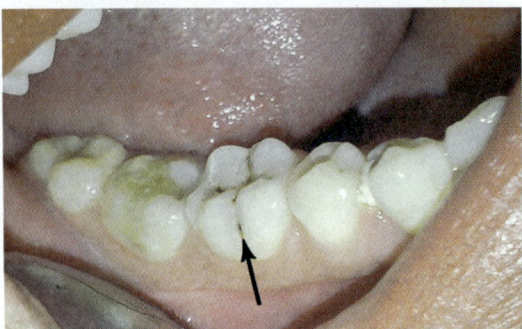

Fig. 2.2: *Pit and fissure caries involving buccal fissure*

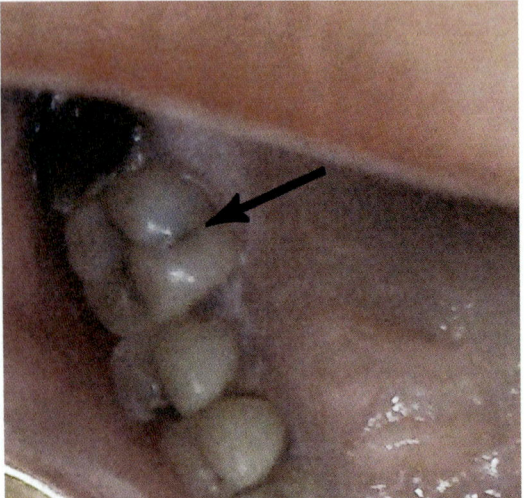

Fig. 2.3: *Pit and fissure caries involving palatal fissure*

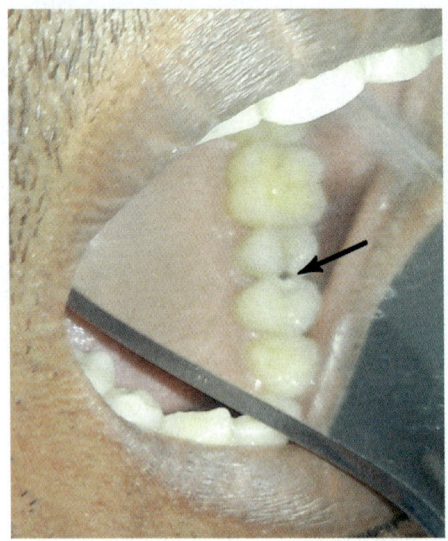

Fig. 2.4: *Smooth surface caries involving proximal surface of posterior tooth*

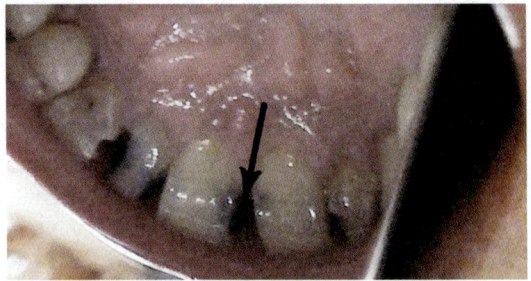

Fig. 2.5: *Smooth surface caries involving proximal surface of anterior tooth*

b. *Smooth surface caries (proximal and cervical caries)*: Caries occurring on smooth surfaces of the teeth (Figs 2.4 to 2.6)

c. *Root caries*: Caries occurring at the cementoenamel junction or cementum. This occurs predominantly in the older age when there is gingival recession (Fig. 2.7).

d. *Linear enamel caries*: Caries occurring on the labial surfaces of anterior teeth. This is also known as '*Odontoclasia*'. The caries occurs at neonatal zone because of trauma at birth or metabolic disturbances.

B. According to Severity of Lesion

a. *Incipient caries*: Incipient caries appears as a white opaque region on any tooth surface.

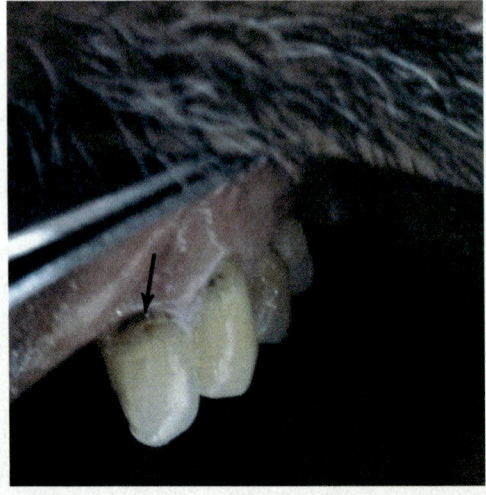

Fig. 2.6: *Smooth surface caries involving cervical part of tooth*

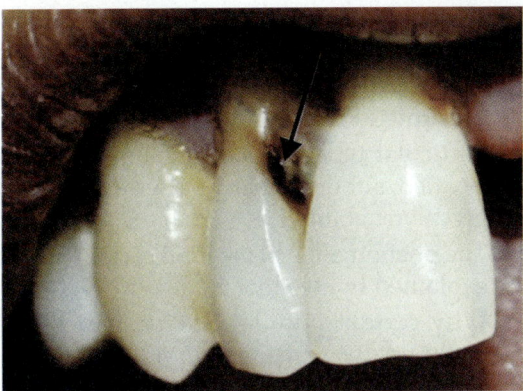

Fig. 2.7: *Root caries*

No major histological change appears, only surface demineralization of enamel occurs. A white lesion or incipient lesion can undergo remineralization thereby reversing the process.

b. *Rampant caries*: It is the sudden and rapid onset of caries involving at least two teeth and two surfaces. A caries increment of ten or more new carious lesions over a year is characteristic of rampant caries.

c. *Radiation caries*: One of the complications of radiotherapy of oral cancer lesions is xerostomia, which leads to an early development of widespread caries.

C. According to Progress of Lesion

a. *Acute caries:* Acute caries implies rapid progress involving large number of teeth.

b. *Chronic caries:* Chronic caries implies slow progress and less number of teeth.

c. *Arrested caries:* Any carious lesion, usually an incipient, may become arrested, if there is a change in oral environment. The arrested caries, clinically appears as a dark brown pigmentation with smooth surface. This is referred to as 'Eburnation'. It can be on occlusal as well as on interproximal surfaces.

D. According to Virginity of Lesion

a. *Primary caries (initial caries):* The initial location of caries is designated as primary caries.

b. *Secondary caries (recurrent caries)*: It occurs at interface of tooth and restorative material because of many factors such as defective cavity preparation, microleakage and combination of these.

E. According to Age Pattern

a. *Nursing bottle caries*: In early infancy period, bottle fed babies develop caries usually on maxillary incisors. The prolonged breast-feeding especially at night can also result in such caries.

b. *Early childhood caries:* Caries occurring during early childhood and pre-school children (2–5 yr).

c. *Adolescent caries:* Caries attack during puberty and teens is usually characterized as adolescent caries.

d. *Geriatric caries*: Caries which occurs in older adults (age 65+) is referred to as geriatric caries.

F. Based on WHO System

The shape and depth of caries is scored on a four point scale:

D1: Clinically detectable enamel lesion with intact (non-cavitated) surface

D2: Clinically detectable lesion limited to enamel

D3: Clinically detectable lesion in dentin

D4: Lesions extending into pulp

ETIOLOGY OF DENTAL CARIES

Dental caries is a multifactorial disease. Till today, no single theory can explain the phenomenon of caries. The caries is not inflammatory in origin nor is it degenerative in nature and neither is it a neoplasm. Dental caries is a local disease, which involves destruction of hard tissues of tooth by metabolites produced by micro-organisms. The theories are:

1. The Worm Theory

The cause of caries was thought to be invasion of 'worms' into teeth. Therefore the character of caries was shown as a worm over tooth surface.

2. The Humoral Theory

The humoral theory implies that the dental caries was produced by internal action of acids and corroding humors. The four recognized humors of the body were blood, phlegm, black bile and yellow bile. The imbalance in these humors resulted in the disease process.

3. Vital Theory

It was postulated that tooth decay originated from within the tooth itself. The authors studied the caries histologically and observed wider area beneath and smaller pinpoint area on top of the tooth.

4. Parasitic Theory

The filamentous parasites in the membrane of tooth surfaces were also considered as the causative agent for dental caries.

5. Acidogenic Theory

Miller (1889) who propagated this concept was of the view that micro-organisms of the oral cavity degrade the carbohydrates into acids (lactic acid, butyric acid, etc.). The acid so produced demineralizes the enamel. Subsequently, demineralized enamel is mechanically removed by the forces of mastication. After the disintegration of enamel, the organisms and acids penetrate dentinal tubules and bring about the dissolution of dentin. The proteolytic enzymes finally digest the organic part.

Miller was of the view that no single species of micro-organisms were capable of producing acids and digesting proteins. His work was confirmed by the following facts:

- Acid was present in the deeper carious lesions.
- Several micro-organisms of oral cavity were capable of producing acids.
- Lactic acid was identified in carbohydrate-saliva combined mixtures.
- Different micro-organisms had the potential to invade carious dentin.

Though Miller's theory is relevant till date as far as caries etiology is concerned, certain points need to be explored further which were not clear with his theory.

- The smooth surface caries was not accounted for in this theory.
- Particular type of micro-organism was not isolated, although many bacteria possessed glycolytic abilities.
- The phenomenon of arrested caries was not explained by this theory.
- Why certain populations are caries-free could not be explained by Miller.
- Caries of un-erupted/impacted teeth was not explained.
- One accepted phenomenon that the carious dentin, if left under a filling continues to decay remained unsolved.

6. Proteolytic Theory

Gottlieb (1944) was of the view that instead of decalcification of inorganic part, the initial action is due to the proteolytic enzymes attacking the organic components.

Caries is initiated at a slightly alkaline pH produced by the proteolytic activity liquefying the organic matrix of enamel. Once the inorganic part sets free after the dissolution of organic part, these salts are dissolved subsequently by acidogenic bacteria.

7. Proteolysis Chelation Theory

The proteolysis chelation theory considers dental caries to be a bacterial destruction of organic component of enamel and the breakdown products of these organic components to have chelating properties and thereby dissolve the minerals in the enamel. It is hypothesized that there is a simultaneous microbial degradation of organic component by proteolysis and the dissolution of inorganic part by the process of chelation. The word 'chelate' refers to compounds that are able to bind metallic ions such as calcium, iron, copper, zinc, etc. by valence bonds

8. Levine's Theory

Levine (1977) emphasized that the demineralization and remineralization of enamel is a continuous process. He hypothesized that minerals move from saliva/plaque to enamel and vice versa, the phenomenon is termed as the ionic 'see-saw' mechanism. If in a given interval of time, more ions leave the enamel than enter it, then there is a net demineralization; subsequently leading to the carious process.

At times, the chemical conditions at enamel-plaque interface may favour outward movement of ions and at other times the situation may be reversed. This delicate balance of ions is dependent on many factors. The three most important factors viz. pH of plaque, calcium and phosphate ion concentration at the interface and fluoride ion concentration are responsible.

If the pH falls below 5, mineral ions are liberated from the hydroxyapatite crystals of the enamel surface and diffuse into plaque. Some of the ions are lost and others are deposited onto the enamel. With such repeated episodes, over all demineralization occurs which may lead to caries. If free calcium and phosphate ions are higher in the saliva, there would be a greater tendency of ions to move from plaque to enamel. Fluoride also favours movement of ions from plaque to enamel.

9. Bandlish's Theory

According to Bandlish oral fluids protect the enamel by providing a protective covering on the enamel surface. Attrition makes the fissures wider and removes the superficial layer of the enamel along with the initial carious lesion, if present. The new layer of enamel becomes protective again with the help of oral fluids. In areas where the oral fluids, cannot reach, e.g. contact areas, enamel cannot be made protective against the carious attack. The effect of acid attack depends upon the perimeter/unit area.

Greater the perimeter, stronger would be the attack. As the length of the perimeter/unit area falls with increase in size of the contact area, the carious lesion progress faster in a smaller contact area, if other conditions are kept constant.

During the buccolingual movement of teeth (proximal surface), there is more movement at the occlusal border of the contact area and less at the cervical border (less movement near the fulcrum). Where there is more movement there is less incidence of caries; where there is less movement there is more incidence of caries. Accordingly, the cervical border of the contact area is more prone to caries.

Meticulous brushing and cleaning reduces caries not by removing plaque but by removing some part of enamel. Plaque acts as a reservoir of minerals and with its buffering capabilities helps in maturation of enamel surface, thereby reducing caries.

In case of occlusal caries, caries starts at places where there is least attrition and least plaque, i.e. where contact of two or more enamel surfaces occurs like in fissures and at cusp tips.

Contributory Factors in Dental Caries

Dental caries is a multi-factorial disease. Caries occur when all the four factors are favourable: that is, susceptible host, cariogenic oral flora, a suitable substrate and sufficient length of time.

The four factors contributing to the caries process are:
1. The host factor
   a. Morphology and chemical nature of teeth
   b. Composition, flow and antibacterial activity of saliva
2. Microflora
3. Substrate or diet
   a. Physical nature
   b. Chemical nature
4. Time

1. The Host Factor

a. *Morphology and chemical nature of teeth*

Deep pits and fissures in any tooth make them susceptible to caries because of food impaction and bacterial stagnation. The most susceptible teeth are the mandibular first molars.

Irregularities in the arch form, crowding and overlapping of the teeth also favour development of caries.

Presence of inorganic constituents (dicalcium phosphate dihydrate, fluoroapatite, etc.) makes the enamel resistant to caries. The outer enamel is more caries resistant than the subsurface enamel because of accumulation of minerals on the outer enamel surface.

b. *Composition, flow and antibacterial activity of saliva*

The flow of saliva affects the oral environment and its effect on dental caries cannot be ruled out. Human beings suffering from decreased flow of saliva or lack of salivary secretions (xerostomia) usually experience increased rate of dental caries.

Caries prone individuals have low calcium and phosphorous levels. The caries immune persons exhibit greater ammonia content in saliva.

The pH at which any saliva ceases to be saturated with calcium and phosphorous is referred to as the 'critical pH'. Under normal conditions the critical pH is 5.5. Below this value, the inorganic material of the tooth may dissolve. The normal pH of resting saliva is 6–7. A buffer is a solution that tends to main-tain a constant pH. A fall in buffer capacity of saliva leads to increase in caries incidence.

Lysozyme, an antibacterial agent present in saliva, can inhibit airborne and waterborne micro-organisms in the oral cavity, but its role in caries inhibition is doubtful. Antibodies like secretory IgA and IgG against specific bacteria have been reported in human saliva.

2. Microflora

Bacteria play a definite role in initiation and progress of caries. The following factors further prove the role of bacteria in caries:

i. Caries will not occur in complete absence of micro-organisms

ii. All oral organisms may not be cariogenic, but majority can be isolated from carious lesions

The experimental studies on caries indicate that different organisms display some selectivity as to which tooth surface they would prefer. There are differences in occlusal caries and root caries and also in smooth surface caries and pit and fissure caries. The main etiological micro-organism in occlusal and pit and fissure caries is the *Streptococcus mutans*.

The predominantly micro-organisms present in deep caries are lactobacilli which account for one-third of the oral flora.

The organisms involved in root caries are different from those in other smooth surface lesions. Predominantly *Actinomyces viscosus* have been isolated. Other species of Actinomyces such as *A. naeslundii* and *Nocardia* etc. have also been isolated.

3. Substrate or Diet

Diet refers to the customary food, which we take from time to time and nutrition means the assimilated portion of diet, which affects the metabolic process of body. Diet has shown to influence caries.

a. Physical Nature of Diet

The raw food leads to attrition and also clean the debris, thereby reduces caries. Modern diet includes refined foods, soft drinks and eatables, which lead to collection of debris predisposing to more caries. Further, it is observed that the mastication of food reduces the number of micro-organisms.

b. Chemical Nature of Diet

Chemical nature of diet implies the nutrients present in our meals and their cariogenic potential. The main ingredient is carbohydrate, which is accepted as one of the most important factor in dental caries process. Only refined carbohydrates are effective. The frequency of intake and time of stagnation of carbohydrates is important.

The vitamin ingredient of diet has also been considered to have significant effect on dental caries incidence. Vitamins A, C and K rarely have any effect on caries production. Vitamin B deficiency may exert a caries protective influence on teeth since several B vitamins are essential in growth of oral acidogenic flora.

Certain minerals such as calcium and phosphorous and trace elements such as selenium and vanadium may influence dental caries. Fluoride in various forms also inhibits caries. It has been proved that fluoride content of caries free teeth is higher than the carious teeth. Fluoride in drinking water within practical limits reduces caries. Use of fluorides in pastes, etc. remained controversial because of ingestion of fluoride especially in young individuals. Topical application of fluoride in a similar way is effective.

4. Time

The frequency of cariogenic environment affecting the teeth is significant in development of caries.

SECONDARY CARIES

Secondary caries can be defined as caries around a restoration. It is also known as 'recurrent caries'. The caries may be present at surface enamel surrounding the restoration or extend underneath it along the margins. Similar to secondary caries is contact caries, which refers to caries on the opposing tooth surface in contact with the restoration. The main etiological factor for secondary caries is marginal leakage around the restorations. Rough enamel surfaces are more susceptible to demineralization than smooth ones. Accordingly, the formation of secondary carious lesions may be higher in unpolished than in polished enamel surfaces.

RESIDUAL CARIES

Caries that remains after the cavity preparation has been completed is referred to as residual caries, which may have been left behind either intentionally by the operator or by accident. Residual caries at the dentino-enamel junction or enamel walls is not acceptable. Only affected dentin can be left behind.

3

Nomenclature and Terminology

Operative dentistry is defined as 'the branch of dentistry which deals with the diagnosis, prognosis, treatment and prevention of defects of the teeth, restoring them to their form, function and esthetics, thereby maintaining the stomatognathic system.'

Before starting with the actual subject, the technical terms used during the treatment along with the nomenclature should be thoroughly understood. Let us first be familiar with the notation systems fall into two categories:

The majority of the tooth notation system falls into two categories:

A. Those having a *similar* notation for the teeth in each segment

B. Those having a *different* notation for the teeth in each segment

A. Systems having a Similar Notation in Each Segment

System I: The oldest known method in this group still in use is probably 'Zsigmondy system'. This is also known as Palmer's Notation. The central incisor of each segment is given the number '1' and the numbers then run in a distal direction. The segments are shown as the patients' upper right, upper left, lower right and lower left segments respectively.

Zsigmondy's system

Permanent teeth

$$R \dfrac{8\ 7\ 6\ 5\ \ 4\ \ 3\ \ 2\ \ 1 \ \ | \ \ 1\ \ 2\ \ 3\ \ 4\ \ 5\ \ 6\ \ 7\ \ 8}{8\ 7\ 6\ 5\ \ 4\ \ 3\ \ 2\ \ 1 \ \ | \ \ 1\ \ 2\ \ 3\ \ 4\ \ 5\ \ 6\ \ 7\ \ 8} L$$

The temporary teeth are indicated merely by replacing the Arabic numerals to Roman ones. Sometimes temporary teeth are designated with letters 'a' – 'e' or with capital letters 'A' – 'E'.

Different variants for temporary teeth

$$R \dfrac{e\ \ d\ \ c\ \ b\ \ a \ \ | \ \ a\ \ b\ \ c\ \ d\ \ e}{e\ \ d\ \ c\ \ b\ \ a \ \ | \ \ a\ \ b\ \ c\ \ d\ \ e} L$$

$$R \dfrac{E\ \ D\ \ C\ \ B\ \ A \ \ | \ \ A\ \ B\ \ C\ \ D\ \ E}{E\ \ D\ \ C\ \ B\ \ A \ \ | \ \ A\ \ B\ \ C\ \ D\ \ E} L$$

System II: The other system does not make use of numerals, but designates the teeth (starting from the central incisor) as:

$I_1, I_2, C, P_1, P_2, M_1, M_2$ and M_3, i.e. the initial letters of their respective Latin names. Temporary teeth are shown with small letters, sometimes supplemented with the letter'd' (deciduous) preceding the letter symbol.

Permanent teeth

$$R \dfrac{M_3\ M_2\ M_1\ P_2\ P_1\ C\ I_2\ I_1\ |\ I_1\ I_2\ C\ P_1\ P_2\ M_1\ M_2\ M_3}{M_3\ M_2\ M_1\ P_2\ P_1\ C\ I_2\ I_1\ |\ I_1\ I_2\ C\ P_1\ P_2\ M_1\ M_2\ M_3} L$$

Primary teeth

$$R \dfrac{dm_2\ dm_1\ dc\ di_2\ di_1\ |\ di_1\ di_2\ dc\ dm_1\ dm_2}{dm_2\ dm_1\ dc\ di_2\ di_1\ |\ di_1\ di_2\ dc\ dm_1\ dm_2} L$$

B. Systems with Different Notation in Each Segment

Several systems which employ different notations for the teeth in different segments are in use. The 'Universal System' is most commonly used.

Universal system (permanent teeth)

$$R \frac{1 \quad 2 \quad 3 \quad 4 \quad 5 \quad 6 \quad 7 \quad 8 \mid 9 \quad 10 \ 11 \ 12 \ 13 \ 14 \ 15 \ 16}{32 \ 31 \ 30 \ 29 \ 28 \ 27 \ 26 \ 25 \mid 24 \ 23 \ 22 \ 21 \ 20 \ 19 \ 18 \ 17} L$$

Universal system (deciduous teeth)

$$R \frac{A \quad B \quad C \quad D \quad E \mid F \quad G \quad H \quad I \quad J}{T \quad S \quad R \quad Q \quad P \mid O \quad N \quad M \quad L \quad K} L$$

The universal system has also a variant employing the letter 'D' for temporary or deciduous teeth as follows:

The universal system

$$R \frac{D1 \quad D2 \quad D3 \quad D4 \quad D5 \mid D6 \quad D7 \quad D8 \quad D9 \quad D10}{D20 \ D19 \ D18 \ D17 \ D16 \mid D15 \ D14 \ D13 \ D12 \ D11} L$$

FDI system: The Federation Dentaire Internationale (FDI)/Two digit system is an accepted system. The notation is as follows:

Permanent teeth

Maxillary

$$R \frac{18 \ 17 \ 16 \ 15 \ 14 \ 13 \ 12 \ 11 \mid 21 \ 22 \ 23 \ 24 \ 25 \ 26 \ 27 \ 28}{48 \ 47 \ 46 \ 45 \ 44 \ 43 \ 42 \ 41 \mid 31 \ 32 \ 33 \ 34 \ 35 \ 36 \ 37 \ 38} L$$

Mandibular

Primary teeth

Maxillary

$$R \frac{55 \ 54 \quad 53 \ 52 \quad 51 \mid 61 \quad 62 \ 63 \quad 64 \ 65}{85 \ 84 \quad 83 \ 82 \quad 81 \mid 71 \quad 72 \ 73 \quad 74 \ 75} L$$

Mandibular

The, FDI two digit system identifies each of the 32 permanent teeth with a two digit number, the first digit indicating the quadrant (1 to 4, starting from upper right quadrant clockwise to lower right quadrant) and the second digit indicating the tooth type (1 to 8, starting from central incisor to the third molar). The 20 primary teeth are represented in a similar fashion: quadrant as 5 to 8 and tooth type as 1 to 5.

The advantages of this system are:
- Simple to teach and understand
- Readily communicable in print and on telephone
- Easy to speak in conversation and dictation
- Easy to enter into a computer
- Easily adaptable to standard charts used in general practice.

Terminology Related to Tooth Surfaces (Table 3.1)

Caries involving any of these surfaces is denoted by that particular surface name used as a prefix before the word 'caries', e.g. Caries on the mesial surface of the tooth is referred to as mesial caries. Caries involving two surfaces say mesial and occlusal is referred to as mesio-occlusal (MO) caries. Caries involving three surfaces say mesial, occlusal and distal is refered to as mesio-occlusodistal (MOD) caries.

Anatomical tooth crown and clinical tooth crown: Portion of the tooth that is covered with enamel is referred to as the anatomical tooth crown. Portion of the tooth that is exposed in the oral cavity is referred to as the clinical tooth crown.

Anatomic tooth root and clinical tooth root: Portion of the tooth that is covered with cementum is referred to as the anatomical tooth root. Portion of the tooth that is not visible in the oral cavity is referred to as the clinical tooth root.

Table 3.1 *Different surfaces of the tooth are named according to their adjoining anatomic structures*

Facial surfaces	Labial surface	• Facing towards the lip
	Buccal surface	• Facing towards the cheek
Lingual surface		• Facing towards the tongue
Palatal surface		• Facing towards the palate
Mesial surface		• Facing towards the midline
Distal surface		• Facing away from the midline
Incisal surface		• Functioning edges of the incisors and canines
Occlusal surface		• Functioning/masticating surfaces of the premolars and molars
Cervical portion		• Portion of the tooth related to the cervical line or necks of teeth
Gingival portion		• Portion of the tooth close to the gingiva

TERMINOLOGY RELATED TO CARIES

The definition and types of caries are given in Chapter 2

Nomenclature Related to Cavity Preparation

Cavity: A cavity in general is a hollow or space within the body or one of its organs. In dentistry, the lesion produced by dental caries is designated as cavity.

Cavity preparation: Cavity preparation is the orderly procedure required to remove diseased tissue and establish a biomechanically acceptable form in the tooth to receive a restorative material such that the tooth is returned to its normal form, function and esthetics (where needed).

Intracoronal preparation: Preparation that involves interior of the tooth is referred to as the intracoronal preparation (inlays and direct restorations).

Extracoronal preparation: Preparation that involves the external surfaces of the tooth which may need removal of part or total enamel is referred to as the extracoronal preparation, e.g. onlays and crown preparation.

Simple Cavities

Cavities involving only one surface of the tooth are called simple cavities, e.g. mesial (M), distal (D), facial (F), lingual (L), occlusal (O) and incisal (I) cavities (Fig. 3.1).

Compound Cavities

Cavities involving two adjoining surfaces of the tooth are called compound cavities (Fig. 3.2), for example:

MO	:	Mesio-occlusal cavity
MB	:	Mesiobuccal cavity
ML	:	Mesiolingual cavity
DO	:	Disto-occlusal cavity
DB	:	Distobuccal cavity
DL	:	Distolingual cavity

Complex Cavities

Cavities involving more than two adjoining surfaces of the tooth are called complex cavities (Fig. 3.3), for example:

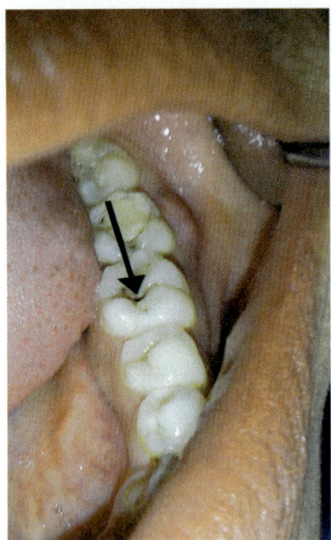

Fig. 3.1: *Caries involving one side (occlusal surface)*

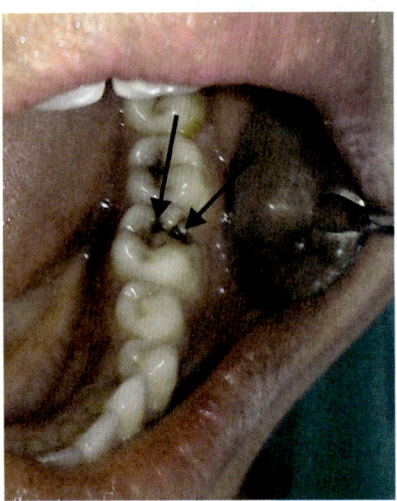

Fig. 3.2: *Caries involving two sides (buccal and occlusal)*

Mesio-occlusodistal cavity (MOD cavity)
Mesioincisodistal cavity (MID cavity)
Facio-occlusolingual cavity (FOL cavity)

Recently, the complex cavities are designated as those cavities which need extra retentive device for their restorations.

Walls in a Cavity Preparation

Wall: Any surface of the cavity is referred to as a wall.

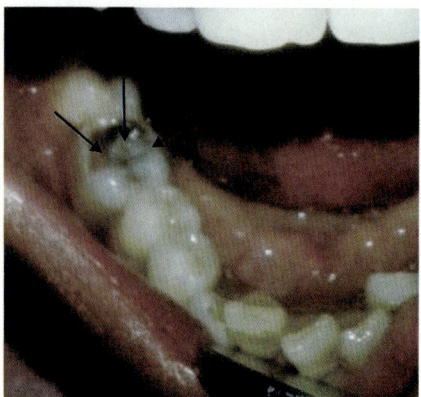

Fig. 3.3: *Caries involving three sides (buccal, occlusal and lingual)*

Internal wall: Surface of a prepared cavity that does not extend to the exterior of the tooth is referred to as an internal wall.

External wall: Surface of a prepared cavity that extends on to the exterior of the tooth is referred to as an external wall.

Enamel wall: That portion of the cavity wall which is composed of enamel is called an enamel wall.

Dentin wall: That portion of the cavity wall which is composed of dentin is called dentin wall.

Floor/seat of the cavity: Any cavity wall that is flat and perpendicular to the forces directed

occlusogingivally is referred to as a floor/seat of the cavity, e.g. pulpal and gingival walls.

Step: An auxiliary extension of the main cavity on to an adjoining surface is referred to as a step, e.g. in a class III cavity with a lingual dovetail, the lingual dovetail is referred to as a lingual step.

Dentinoenamel Junction (DEJ): The line of union between enamel and dentin is referred to as the dentinoenamel junction.

Cementoenamel Junction (CEJ): The line of union between enamel and cementum is referred to as the cementoenamel junction.

Different walls of the cavity are named according to the surfaces towards which they face (Table 3.2).

Walls in an Occlusal Cavity (Class I, Fig. 3.4)

• Facial wall
• Lingual wall
• Mesial wall
• Distal wall
• Pulpal wall

Walls in a Proximo-occlusal Cavity (Class II, Fig. 3.5)

Occlusal portion

• Facial wall
• Lingual wall

Table 3.2: *Different walls of the cavity are faced according to the surface*	
Facial surfaces < Labial surface	• Wall facing towards the lips
Buccal surface	• Facing towards the cheek
Lingual surface	• Facing towards the tongue
Lingual/palatal walls	• Walls facing towards the tongue and palate respectively
Incisal/occlusal walls	• Walls facing towards the incisal and occlusal portions of the tooth respectively
Mesial/distal walls	• Walls facing towards the mesial and distal aspects of the tooth respectively
Axial wall	• Wall nearest the pulp and parallel to the long axis of the tooth in cavities present on the axial surfaces
Pulpal wall	• Wall nearest the pulp and perpendicular to the long axis of the tooth in cavities present on the occlusal surface or incisal edges of the teeth
Gingival wall	• Wall facing the gingiva
Subpulpal wall	• When the pulp chamber is accessed and the roof of the pulp chamber removed, the floor of the pulp chamber left behind is referred to as the subpulpal wall

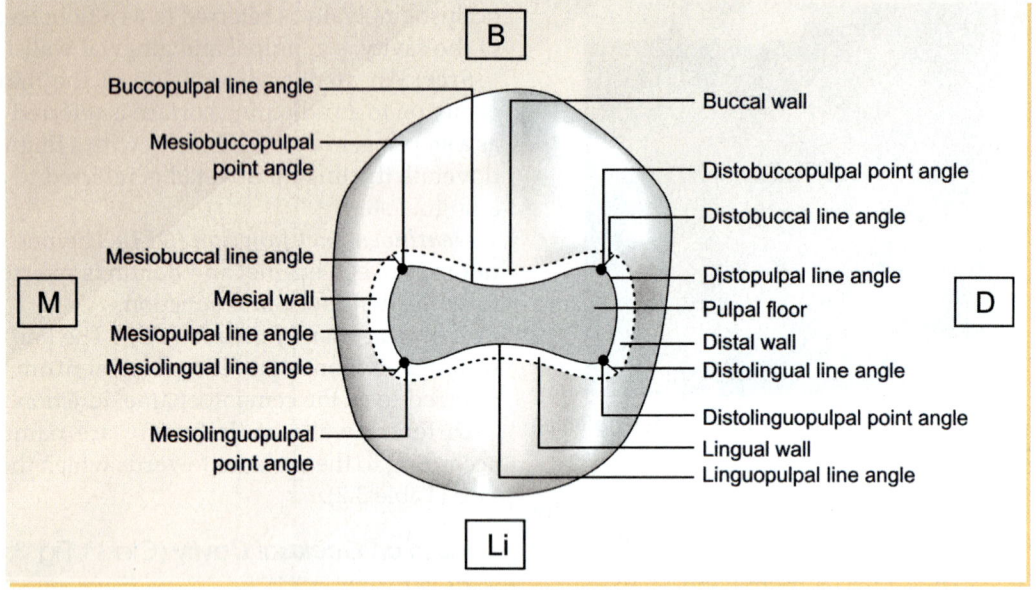

Fig. 3.4: *Walls and angles in an occlusal class I cavity*

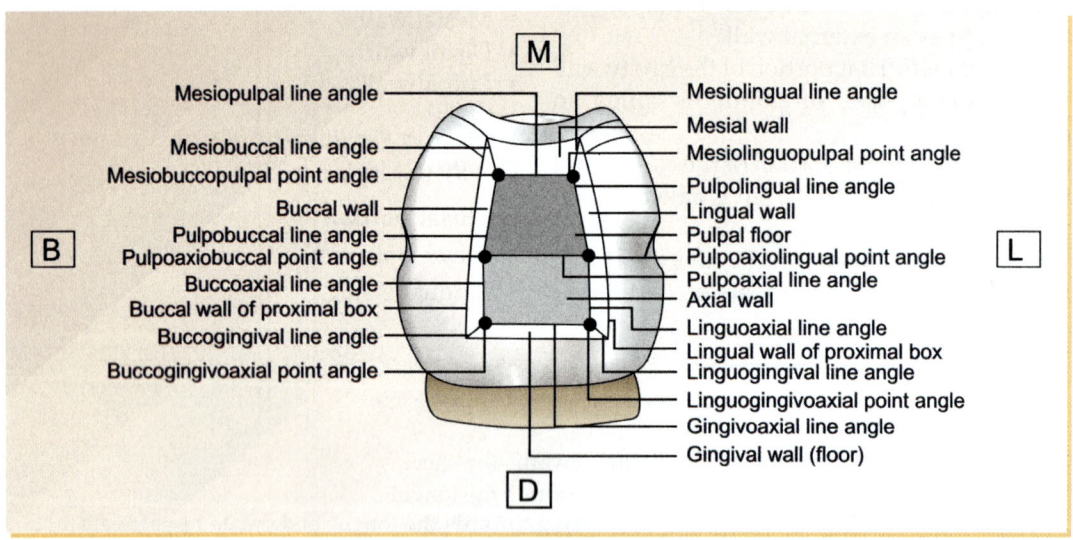

Fig. 3.5: *Walls and angles in a class II cavity*

- Mesial or distal wall (any one of these, depending on which surface the cavity is present)
- Pulpal wall

Proximal portion
- Facioproximal wall
- Linguoproximal wall
- Gingival wall
- Axial wall

Walls in a Proximal Cavity (Class III, Fig. 3.6)
- Facial wall
- Lingual wall
- Gingival wall
- Axial wall

Walls in a Proximal Incisal Cavity (Class IV)

Incisal step
- Facial wall
- Lingual wall

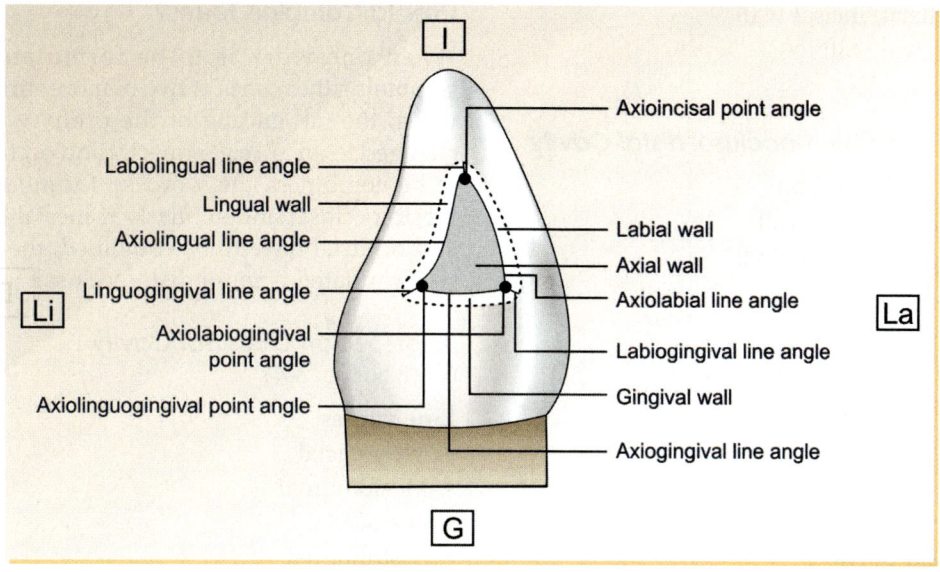

Fig. 3.6: *Walls and angles in a class III cavity*

- Mesial or distal wall (any one of these depending on which surface the cavity is present)
- Pulpal wall

Proximal portion

- Facioproximal wall
- Linguoproximal wall

- Gingival wall
- Axial wall

Walls in Facial and Lingual Cavities (Class V, Fig. 3.7)

- Mesial wall
- Distal wall

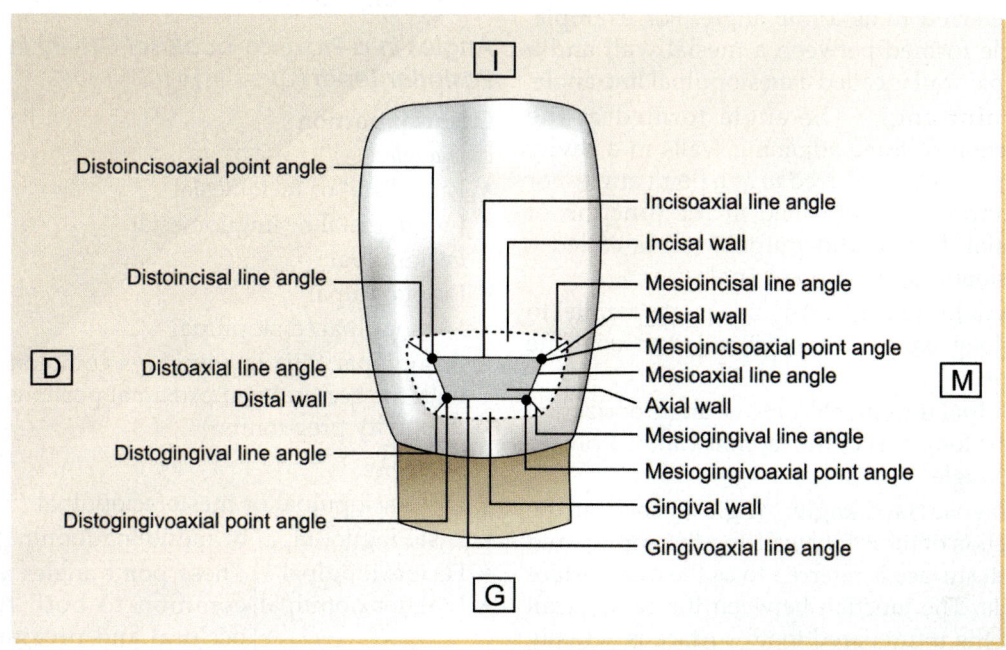

Fig. 3.7: *Walls and angles in a class V cavity*

- Occlusal/incisal wall
- Gingival wall
- Axial wall

Walls in a Mesio-occluso-distal Cavity

Mesial proximal box
- Facioproximal wall
- Linguoproximal wall
- Gingival wall
- Axial wall

Distal proximal box
- Facioproximal box
- Linguoproximal wall
- Gingival wall
- Axial wall

Occlusal portion
- Facial wall.
- Lingual wall
- Pulpal wall

Angles in a Cavity Preparation

Angle: Junction of two or more surfaces of a prepared cavity is designated as angle.

Line angle: The angle formed at the junction of two adjoining walls in a cavity preparation is referred to as a line angle. For example, angle formed between a mesial wall and a pulpal wall is called a mesiopulpal line angle.

Point angle: The angle formed at the junction of three adjoining walls in a cavity preparation is referred to as a point angle. For example, angle formed at the junction of mesial, buccal and pulpal wall is called a mesiobuccopulpal point angle.

Axial line angle: Any line angle parallel to the long axis of the tooth is called an axial line angle.

Pulpal line angel: Any line angle horizontal to the long axis of the tooth is called a pulpal line angle.

Cavosurface angle: Angle formed at the junction of the cavity wall and the unprepared tooth surface is referred to as the cavosurface angle. The junction between the cavity wall and the unprepared tooth surface is actually referred to as the cavosurface margin.

How to Combine Terms?

When one work is to be formulated by combining the names of two or more surfaces/walls, the 'al' ending of the prefix word is changed to an 'o', e.g. if mesial and occlusal is to be combined, the word so formulated is mesio-occlusal and similarly if mesial, distal and occlusal have to be combined, the word so formulated is mesiodisto-occlusal.

Angles in an Occlusal Cavity
(Class I, Fig. 3.4)

Line angles
- Mesiofacial
- Mesiolingual
- Distofacial
- Distolingual
- Faciopulpal
- Linguopulpal
- Mesiopulpal
- Distopulpal

Point angles
- Mesiofaciopulpal
- Distofaciopulpal
- Mesiolinguopulpal
- Distolinguopulpal

Angles in a Proximo-occlusal Cavity in Posterior Teeth (Class II, Fig. 3.5)

Occlusal portion
Line angles
- Faciodistal or faciomesial
- Linguodistal or linguomesial
- Faciopulpal
- Linguopulpal
- Mesiopulpal/distopulpal
- Axiopulpal (this line angle is common to both the occlusal and proximal portions of the cavity preparation)

Point angles
- Distofaciopulpal or mesiofaciopulpal
- Distolinguopulpal or mesiolinguopulpal
- Facioaxiopulpal ⎫ These point angles are
- Linguoaxiopulpal ⎬ common to both the occlusal and proximal ⎭ portions of the cavity

Proximal portion

Line angles

- Faciogingival
- Linguogingival
- Facioaxial
- Linguoaxial
- Axiogingival

Point angles

- Faciogingivoaxial
- Linguogingivoaxial

Angles in a Proximal Cavity
(Class III, Fig. 3.6)

Line angles

- Faciogingival
- Linguogingival
- Facioaxial
- Linguoaxial
- Axiogingival
- Faciolingual (incisal)

Point angles

- Facioaxiogingival
- Linguoaxiogingival
- Faciolinguoaxial (incisoaxial)

Angles in a Proximoincisal Cavity in Anterior Teeth *(Class IV)*

Incisal step

Line angles

- Faciomesial or faciodistal
- Linguomesial or linguodistal
- Faciopulpal
- Linguopulpal
- Mesiopulpal or distopulpal
- Axiopulpal (this line angle is common to both the incisal and proximal portion of the cavity preparation).

Point angles

- Faciomesiopulpal or faciodistopulpal
- Linguomesiopulpal or linguodistopulpal
- Facioaxiopulpal ⎫ These point angles are
- Linguoaxiopulpal ⎬ common to both the incisal and proximal portions of the cavity ⎭

Proximal portion

Line angles

- Facioaxial
- Linguoaxial
- Faciogingival
- Linguogingival
- Axiogingival

Point angles

- Faciogingivoaxial
- Linguogingivoaxial

Angles in Buccal and Lingual Cavities
(Class V, Fig.3.7)

Line angles

- Mesio-occlusal/Mesioincisal
- Disto-oclusal/Distoincisal
- Mesiogingival
- Distogingival
- Occlusoaxial/Incisoaxial
- Gingivoaxial
- Mesioaxial
- Distoaxial

Point angles

- Mesio-occlusoaxial/Mesioincisoaxial
- Disto-occlusoaxial/Distoincisoaxial
- Mesiogingivoaxial
- Distogingivoaxial

Angles in Mesio-occlusodistal Cavity
(MOD Cavity)

Mesial proximal box

Line angles

- Facioaxial
- Linguoaxial
- Faciogingival
- Linguogingival
- Axiogingival
- Axiopulpal (this line angle is common to the occlusal and proximal portion of the cavity preparation).

Point angles

- Facioaxiogingival
- Linguoaxiogingival
- Facioaxiopulpal ⎫ These point angles are
  ⎬ common to both the
- Linguoaxiopulpal ⎪ occlusal and proximal
  ⎪ portions of the cavity
  ⎭ preparation

Distal Proximal Box

Line angles
- Facioaxial
- Linguoaxial
- Faciogingival
- Linguogingival
- Axiogingival
- Axiopulpal (this line angle is common to both the occlusal and proximal portions of the cavity preparation)

Point angles
- Facioaxiogingival
- Linguoaxiogingival
- Facioaxiopulpal ⎫ These point angles are
- Linguoaxiopulpal ⎬ common to both the occlusal and proximal portions of the cavity preparation

Occlusal portion

Line angles
- Facioaxiopulpal ⎫ These point angles are
- Linguoaxiopulpal ⎬ common to both the occlusal and proximal portions of the cavity preparation

CLASSIFICATION OF CAVITIES

Dr GV Black's classification of cavities conceived in 1895 is still being widely used and is universally accepted. Though Black originally divided the lesions in five categories; Simon later added the sixth.

The cavity classification is as follows:

Class I: Cavities beginning in the anatomical pits and fissures; viz. occlusal surfaces of premolars and molars, the occlusal two-thirds of the buccal and lingual surfaces of the molars, the lingual surfaces of incisors and any other aberrant locations.

Class II: Cavities on the proximal surfaces of premolars and molars.

Class III: Cavities on the proximal surfaces of incisors and canines, but not involving the incisal angle.

Class IV: Cavities on the proximal surfaces of incisors and canines and also involving the incisal angle.

Class V: Cavities on the gingival third of facial and lingual surfaces of all the teeth.

Simon later added a sixth category as follows:

Class VI: Cavities on the incisal edges and cusp tips of all the teeth.

4

Separators, Retainer-Matrices and Wedges

Each human tooth is attached in the alveolar bone socket with fine periodontal fibers. These fibers act as cushion for the underlying supporting bone. Each crown has a definite relationship with adjacent tooth, having respective curves and contours.

Failure to respect and preserve these relationships will not only cause premature failure of the restoration but also periodontal problems as well as initiation of caries around the adjacent tooth structure. A clear understanding of this interproximal relationship will help the clinician to preserve these structures in a much better manner.

The most important function of the proximal contact is the protection of the interdental papillae. On anterior teeth where the papillae form cone-like projections, properly placed point contacts are necessary. A broader buccolingually contacting area is required on bicuspids because the crests of the papillae broaden out in this region. Similarly, as we move distally, the widest contacting area is required on molars because they have the widest interproximal papillae.

Improper configuration of the proximal area may:

i. Cause displacement of teeth buccally, lingually, mesially or distally

ii. Exert a lifting force on the tooth when placed too high occlusally

iii. Disturb the axial relationship of the teeth, resulting in trauma

iv. Cause rotation of the teeth

v. Cause injury to the investing structures by excessively opening or closing the contact and interproximal embrasures

vi. Disturb the coordination of the inclined planes and cusps, causing defective occlusal contacts

vii. Cause vertical or horizontal food impaction.

Tooth Separators

The separation of the teeth is necessary in many situations like:

• For examination of interproximal spaces
• For preparation of cavities
• For insertion and polishing of restorations
• For removal of foreign bodies, such as fruit seeds, fragments of toothpicks, or bone sequestrums, etc.

Two methods are generally employed for accomplishing separation:

a. Slow separation
b. Rapid or immediate separation

a. Slow Separation

In this method, the teeth are slowly and gradually forced apart inserting certain materials between them. The advantage of slow separation is that the repositioning occur physiologically without injuring periodontal ligament fibers. The disadvantage of this method is that the procedure is time consuming and may require many visits.

Materials used for slow separation are base plate, gutta-percha, orthodontic wire, wood or rubber.

b. Rapid or Immediate Separation

This is the most valuable and frequently used method. The rapid separator should carefully be applied and skillfully handled to produce desired results. Though, the method is quick and useful in clinical conditions, yet it may rupture the periodontal ligament fibers causing pain. The rapid or immediate separation is achieved following two principles, viz. Wedge principle and Traction principle.

The separation by 'Wedge principle' is accomplished by the insertion of a pointer wedge shaped device between teeth in order to create space at the contact area. The more the wedges move facially or lingually, the greater will be the separation. This is brought about by mechanical device (Elliot separator) and wedges.

i. *Elliot separator:* Care must be exercised during its fitting to prevent slipping. This type of separation is useful in examining a proximal surface or in final polishing of the contact point after all other contouring has been completed.

ii. *Separation by wedges:* Following type of wedges help in achieving separation:

  a. Wooden wedges

  b. Celluloid or plastic wedges

The separation by 'Traction principle' is accomplished by an instrument, which engages the proximal surfaces of the tooth by means of holding arms. These are mechanically moved apart, creating separation between the clamped teeth.

The routinely used separators, which work on traction principle, are:

- Non-interfering true separator
- Ferrier double bow separator

Non-interfering true separator: This device is indicated when continuous stabilized separation is required during the dental procedure. Its advantage is that the separation can be increased or decreased after stabili-

zation, and the device is non-interfering (Fig. 4.1).

Ferrier double-bow separator: With this device, the separation is stabilized throughout the procedure. Its advantage is that the separation is shared by the contacting teeth, and not at the expense of one tooth, as with the previous type of instrument (Fig. 4.2).

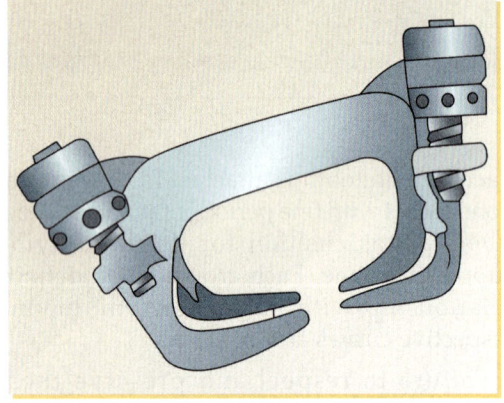

Fig. 4.1: *Non-interfering true separator*

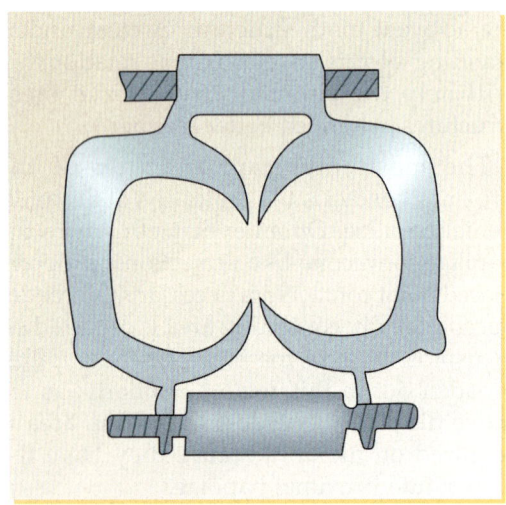

Fig. 4.2: *Ferrier double bow separator*

Matrices

The word matrix is derived from the Latin word 'Mater' which means 'Mother'. The matrix is a device used to contour the proximal/cervical restoration to simulate that of a tooth contours.

Matricing is the procedure, whereby a temporary wall is created opposite to axial walls and surrounding areas of tooth structure that were lost during preparation. Not only should it be immobile while the material sets but also it should not react with it. It should be easily removable after hardening of restorative material without compromising the created contact and contour.

Ideal Requirements

- It should be inserted easily and should be sufficiently rigid to retain the contour given to it so that it can be transferred to the restoration.
- It should not adhere or react with the restorative material.
- It should resist the condensation pressure.

Objectives

- It must act as a temporary wall of resistance during introduction of the restorative material.
- It should provide shape to the restoration.
- It should confine the restoration within acceptable physiological limits.
- It must assist in isolating the gingiva and rubber dam during introduction of the restorative material.
- It must help in maintaining the dry operative field thereby preventing contamination of the restoration.

Classification of Matrices

Matrices are classified in two ways; one is based on mode of retention and second is based on transparency. The retention based matrices are:
- Mechanically retained matrices
- Self-retained matrices

The transparency based matrices are:
- Non-transparent matrices
- Transparent matrices

Materials used as matrices include stainless steel, cellulose acetate (cellophane), cellulose nitrate (celluloid) and polymer materials. Matrix system is formed of two parts; a band, which is made up of either a piece of metal, polymeric material or celluloid and a retainer. Matrices are commonly supplied as strips of different dimensions. They may be 0.001" (0.025 mm) or 0.002" (0.05 mm) thick. The width of the matrix band may be ¼", ⅜", ⁵⁄₁₆" or ⅛".

Depending on the height of the restoration, suitable matrix band is selected. Matrices are also supplied as crown forms, split crown forms and hollow cylinders.

Matrices for Class II, MOD and Complex Restorations

Earlier matrices were not flexible and their insertion around the tooth was difficult (Fig. 4.3). Presently stainless steel matrices of 0.002 inch thicknesses (screwed with the help of retainers) are commonly used. The disadvantages of early matrices were eliminated since the new matrices could be contoured according to the contour of the tooth to be restored.

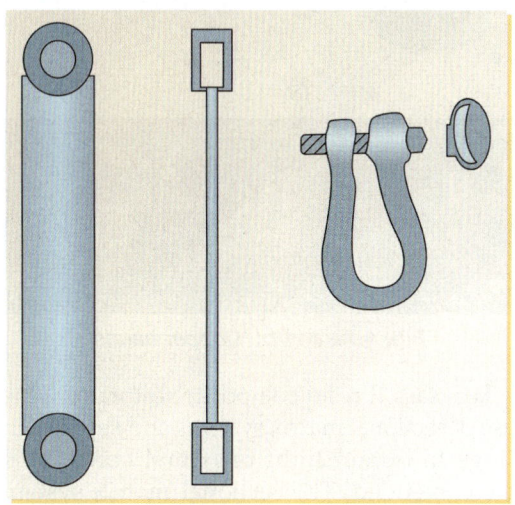

Fig. 4.3: *Loop matrix*

Recently, the demand for rigid type of matrix has been increased because of the use of condensable restorative materials. Such matrices can better withstand the forces of condensation.

A few authors are of the opinion that the matrix be held without the use of retainers, only wedges are sufficient. The rationale is that the retained matrices usually produce straighter proximal areas and matrix held with only wedges produce better contours and contacts.

For MOD preparation and complex restoration, a continuous matrix band is indicated. Such a matrix band may be retained with a mechanical holder and may be ligated. Copper bands can be used for such purposes. These can be trimmed with scissors, smoothened and placed onto the teeth. These can be kept there till the restoration sets. These are mostly used with silver amalgam restorations involving more than two surfaces (Fig. 4.4a and b).

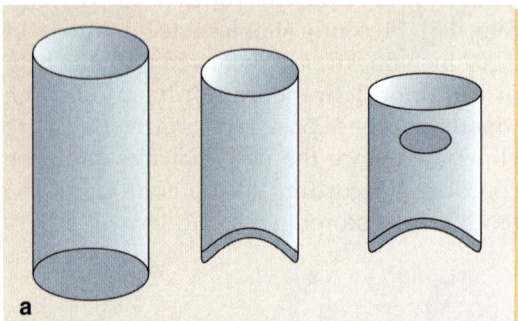

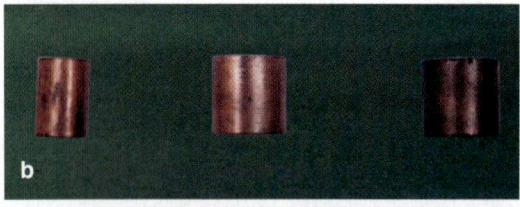

Fig. 4.4a and b: *Copper bands*

For class II resin composite restoration, the use of sectional matrix systems and separation rings to obtain tight proximal contacts is recommended. The sectional matrix system and separation rings are made up of nickel-titanium alloys to create a consistent force to separate teeth and then deliver a tight gingival seal and anatomically shaped restoration. Some of the commercially available systems are:

  i. Palodent Plus sectional matrix system
 ii. Composi-Tight 3D sectional matrix system
iii. Triodent V3 ring matrix system

Matrices for Direct Tooth-colored Restorations

a. Class III Preparations

These are usually transparent plastic matrix strips. For silicate cements (not commonly used) celluloid strips and for resins cellophane strips are used. Mylar strips can be used for both.

The suitable plastic strip is burnished over the end of a steel instrument, e.g. handle of a tweezer, to produce a 'belly' in the strip. This will allow for a curvature, which, if properly contoured and designed, will reproduce the natural proximal contour of the tooth (Fig. 4.5).

In distal surface of canine, since the fixation of retainer is difficult, a metal band is moulded into "S" shape and stabilized using wedges and/or impression compound (Fig. 4.6).

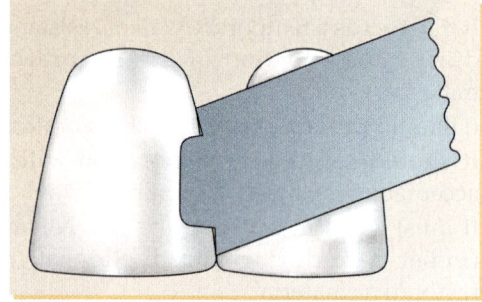

Fig. 4.5: *Matrix for class III preparation*

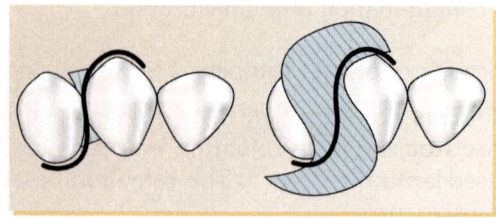

Fig. 4.6: *S-shaped matrix for distal surface of canine*

b. Class IV Preparations

A suitable plastic strip is folded and molded into L shape. One side of the strip is cut so that it is as wide as the length of the tooth. The other side is cut so that it is as wide as the width of the tooth. The strip, with a wedge in place, is adapted to the tooth. It is important that the angle formed by the fold of the strip approximate the normal corner of the tooth and supports the matrix on the lingual surface, which is held by the forefinger of the left hand. The cavity is then filled to slight excess, and one end of the strip is brought across the proximal surface of the filler tooth. When this is completed, the other end of the strip is folded over the incisal edge. The matrix is held with the thumb of the left hand.

Prefabricated matrices are also available. The commonly used are:

i. *Aluminium foil incisal corner matrix:* These are 'stock' metallic matrices shaped according to the proximoincisal corner and surfaces of anterior teeth. This type of matrix cannot be used for light cured resin material (Fig. 4.7).

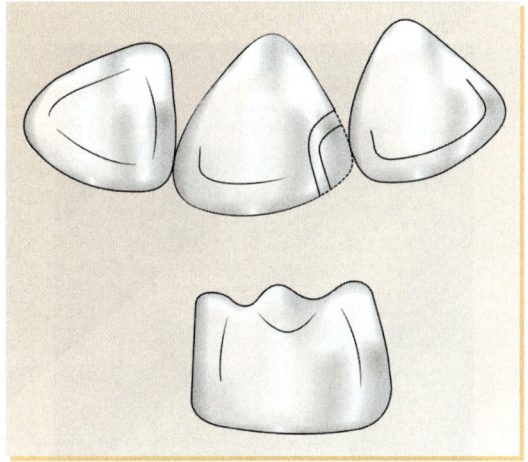

Fig. 4.7: *Matrix for class IV preparation*

ii. *Transparent crown for matrices:* These are 'stock' plastic crowns, which can be adapted to tooth anatomy. In bilateral class IV preparations use the entire crown form; but in a unilateral class IV cut the plastic crown incisogingivally into two halves and use only the side corresponding to the location of the preparation (Fig. 4.8).

iii. *Anatomic matrix:* Prior to preparing the teeth (tooth), a study cast for the affected tooth or teeth along with at least one intact adjacent tooth on each side is made. It is preferable in multiple restorations.

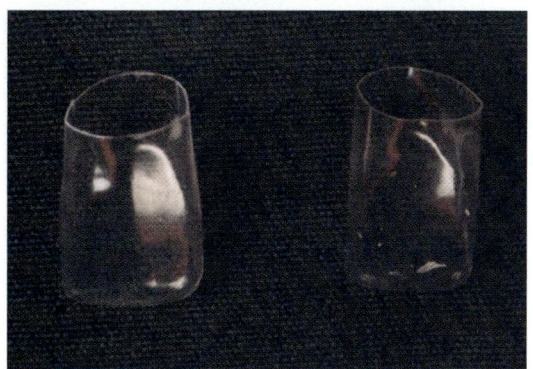

Fig. 4.8: *Transparent celluloid crowns*

The defective areas are restored on the study model in a fairly heat resistant material (plaster, acrylic resin). A plastic template is then made for the restored tooth or teeth on the model using a combination of heat (thermoplastically soften the template material) and suction (vacuum), consequently to draw the moldable material onto the study model. The template is trimmed gingivally so as to seat on at least one unprepared tooth on each side. The restorative material is inserted into the preparation, and then the matrix is filled with the material and inserted over the prepared and partially filled tooth.

c. Class V Preparations

The matrices for class V restorations are available as prefabricated or can be fabricated outside the oral cavity. The commonly available matrices are:

i. *Pefabricated plastic matrices:* These are available in different sizes and can be utilized with light cure restorations. A handle is also provided to hold the matrix in place till the material sets (Fig. 4.9).

ii. *Aluminium or copper collars for non-light cured restorations:* Aluminium or copper bands are preshaped according to the gingival third of the buccal and lingual surfaces. They are adjusted in such a way that the band will cover 1.0–2.0 mm of the tooth surface circumferentially. They are then mounted on the tip of a softened stick of the compound, which is used as a handle. Fill the cavity with restorative

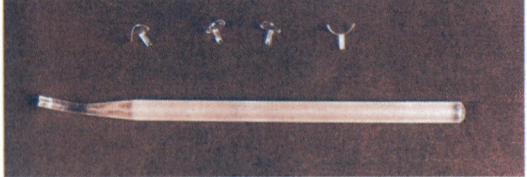

Fig. 4.9: *Matrix for cervical (classs V) preparation*

material and apply the adjusted collar onto the tooth.

iii. *Anatomic matrix for light and non-light cured, direct tooth-colored materials:* Anatomic matrix can be fabricated as for class IV cavities. The study model for the defective tooth or teeth with at least one intact tooth on each side is made. After restoring the defects on the model, a plastic template is prepared. The template is cut mesio-distally, keeping its occlusal (incisal) portion and the facial and lingual parts where the defects are. It is then trimmed gingivally and used as a matrix.

Retainers

The retainers are gadgets used to retain the matrix in position. Some matrices do not need any special mechanical devices to hold them in position. Some matrices may require wires, silk thread, dental floss and impression compound. Some matrices need special mechanical retainers.

The commonly used retainers are:

a. *Ivory matrix holder no. 1 and 8:* The Ivory no.1 is used for class II cavities (Fig. 4.10). Ivory no. 8 provides bands for encircling entire crown of the tooth (Fig. 4.11). This is suitable for both class II cavities and for mesio-occlusodistal cavities. Since the matrix metal is thin enough, it will pass through the contact of the uncut side in the building of the class II amalgam restorations.

b. *The Tofflemire universal matrix retainer:* The Tofflemire retainer (Fig. 4.12) is very stable and permits the easy removal of the holder from the band, facilitating carving and final removal of the band. The retainer is operated as follows:

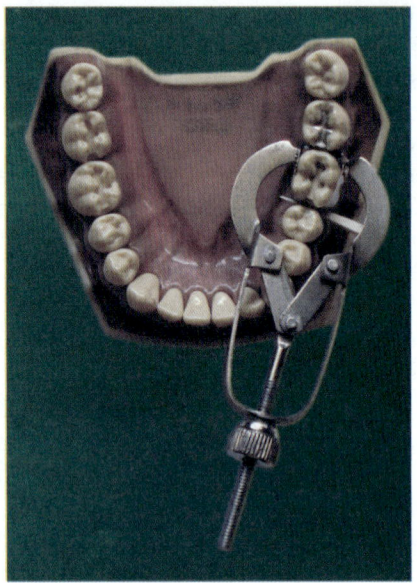

Fig. 4.10: *Application of Ivory no. 1 retainer*

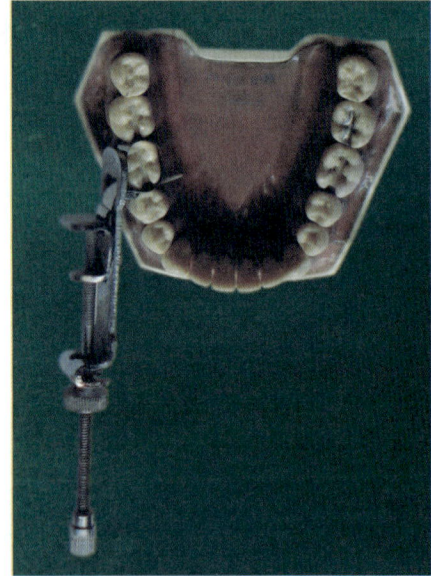

Fig. 4.11: *Application of Ivory no.8 retainer*

• Turn the knurled nut (B) to the right until the diagonal slot (C) is about ¼ inch from the inner end of the diameter (Fig. 4.13a and b).

• Hold the knurled nut (B) from rotating while the knurled nut (A) (at the end of the spindle) is turned a like number of turns in the opposite direction (left), until

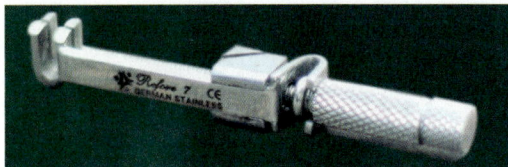

Fig. 4.12a: *Application of Tofflemire retainer*

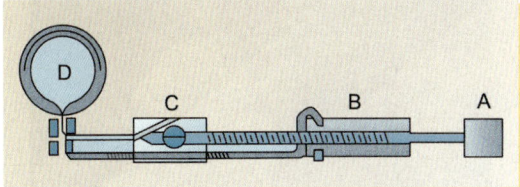

Fig. 4.12b: *Application of Tofflemire retainer (A: knurled nut at the end of the spindle, B: knurled nut, C: diagonal slot, D: matrix band)*

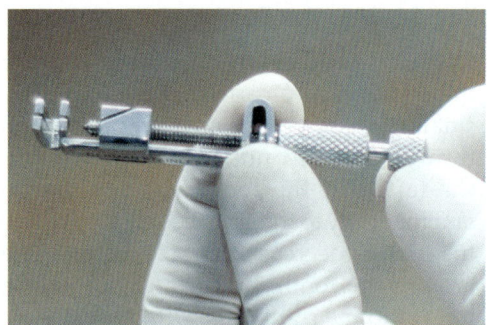

Fig. 4.14: *Hold the knurled nut B from rotating while knurled nut A is turned in opposite direction*

- Insert the 'occlusal edge' of whichever type of matrix band (D) is decided upon in the diagonal slot (C), the preshaped loop, thus formed, is placed in the guide channel selected in such a manner that the metal arch of the guide channel serves as an occlusal 'stop' and materially aids the carrying of the band over the contour of the tooth (Fig. 4.15a and b)

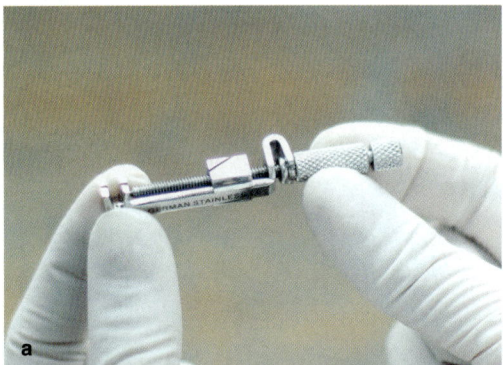

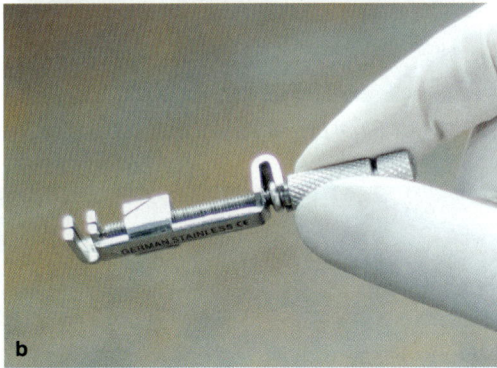

Fig. 4.13a and b: *(a) Turn the knurled nut B to the right, (b) Slot C is about one fourth inch from inner end of the diameter*

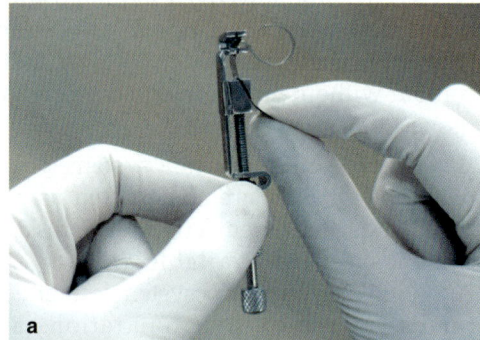

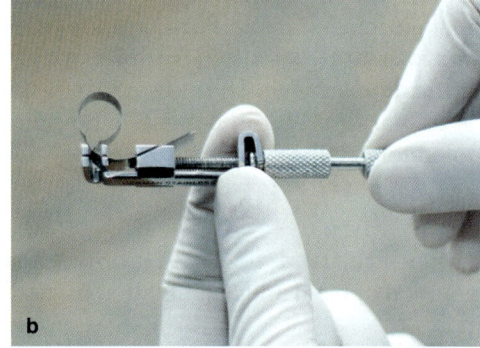

Fig. 4.15a and b: *(a) Insert matrix band D in diagonal slot C, (b) Tighten the band by rotating nut A*

the point of the spindle clears the diagonal slot channel for the reception of the free ends of the matrix band (Fig. 4.14).

Fitting Band to the Teeth

- Guide the band gently over the tooth, using the retainers as a carrier. If the loop is too small to pass over the contour of the tooth, turn the knurled nut (B) a turn or two to the left, and the loop will be enlarged automatically to the size needed. Conversely, the loop is decreased in size, or tightened around the tooth, by turning the knurled nut (B) to the right (Fig. 4.16).

- After restoration, the retainer is removed from the band without disturbing the band.

- The band is then removed carefully from each contact point. Gently ease each interproximal portion of the band out of its inclined plane by using a lateral rotation motion rather than an occlusal traction motion.

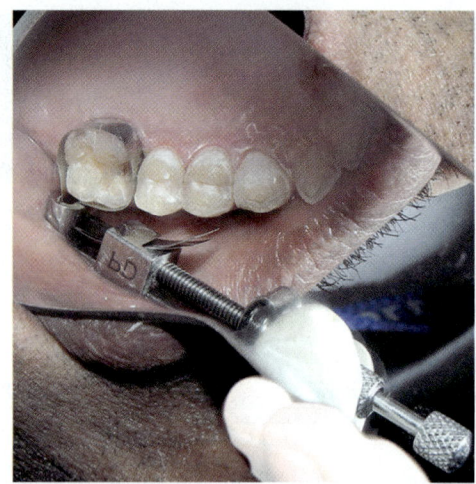

Fig. 4.16a: *Adjust the size of loop according to tooth size by rotating nut B*

c. *Steele's Siqveland self-adjusting matrix:* It is build in such a way that forms two diameters of the band at the same time; larger diameter for the occlusal end and smaller for the gingival end. Anatomic adaptation is possible without wedges, although additional support at the gingival area is not contraindicated. The band follows the tooth contour without impinging on the gingival tissue.

d. *Autonatrix:* Automatrix is a system where band and retainer are constructed as one unit. Bands of different lengths, widths and thicknesses are available (Fig. 4.17). Although the automatrix system is intended for use where cavity preparations are extensive, the instability of this system renders it less suitable. Furthermore, proper contour and proximal contact may be difficult to achieve. The automatrix system is primarily useful in patients who cannot tolerate metallic retainers.

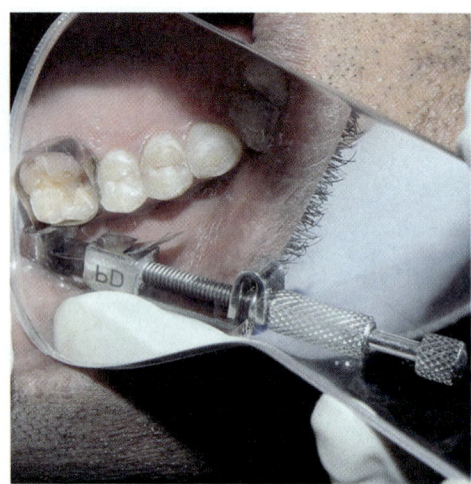

Fig. 4.16b: *Final placement of matrix band system*

Wedges

Wedges are used to bring about rapid separation of teeth and stabilization of matrix band.

Wedging serves the following purposes:

- Prevents surplus amalgam being forced into the gingival crevice.

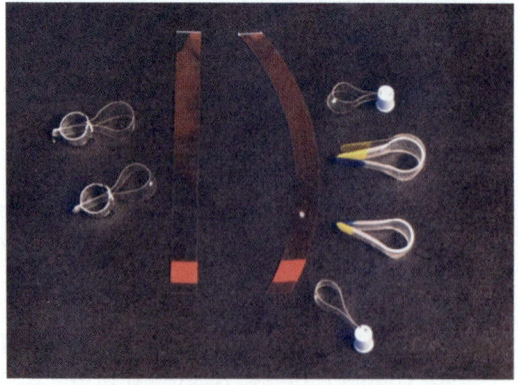

Fig. 4.17: *Automatrix system*

- Assists in contouring the cervical part of the proximal surface.
- Separates the teeth to compensate for the thickness of the matrix band such that proximal contacts are re-established when the band is removed.
- Stabilizes the matrix.

Classification

a. *Wooden or plastic wedges:* Wedges are made of wood or plastic. Wooden wedges are preferred because:
   - They are easy to trim. They adapt well to the tooth surface.
   - They remain stable during condensation.

b. *Preformed or custom made wedges:* Preformed wedges are commercially available in different sizes and are preferred because of their convenience of use.

   The requisite size of custom made wedges may be fabricated from tooth picks.

c. *Triangular (anatomic) or round wedges:* In general a wedge must be triangular or round in cross-section (Fig. 4.18). The width of the base should be slightly larger than the cervical embrasure. If the wedge is not high enough, only point contact between the wedge and the band is achieved. This may lead to poor contour or displacement of the wedge during condensation. A uniform tapering of the wedge is needed in order to render sufficient and even contact throughout the proximal embrasure.

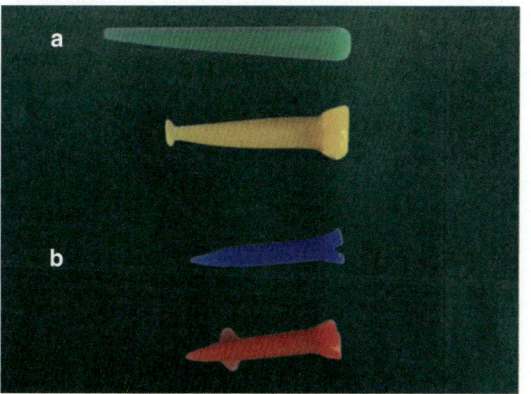

Fig. 4.18: *Wedges*

d. *Opaque or transparent:* Transparent (resin) wedges can be used during placement of composite resin restorations as they allow visible curing light to pass through.

Placement of Wedges

In general, the wedge is inserted from the lingual, as this embrasure is normally larger in size. However, since the lingual wedge will interfere with the tongue, it is preferred form the buccal side. In case of maxillary teeth, placement of wedge is preferred from palatal side. During insertion, care should be taken to ensure that the wedge is apically positioned in relation to the gingival cavity wall.

The clinician should have an adequate knowledge of the anatomical and functional aspects of contacts and contours so as to reproduce them with different restorative materials.

Wedging Systems

1. *'Piggyback' wedging:* If the wedge is significantly apical of the gingival margin, a second, usually smaller wedge may be 'piggybacked' on the first wedge. 'Piggyback' wedging is particularly useful in patients with recession of interproximal area (Fig. 4.19a).

2. *Wedge wedging system:* Occasionally, a concavity may be present on the proximal surface gingivally of the contact and extending as fluting onto the root (e.g. mesial of the maxillary first premolar). A gingival margin located in this area will be similarly concave. To wedge a matrix band tight against such a margin, a second pointed wedge can be inserted between the first wedge and the band by 'wedge wedging'. The wedging action between the teeth should provide enough separation to compensate for the thickness of the matrix band (Fig. 4.19b).

3. *Double wedging system:* In teeth with faciolingually wide proximal boxes, traditionally double wedging has been proposed. It refers to insertion of wedges-

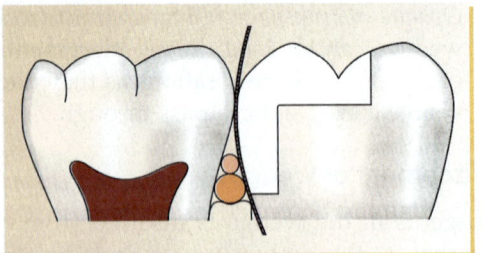

Fig. 4.19a: *Piggyback wedging: Smaller wedge may be piggybacked on first wedge*

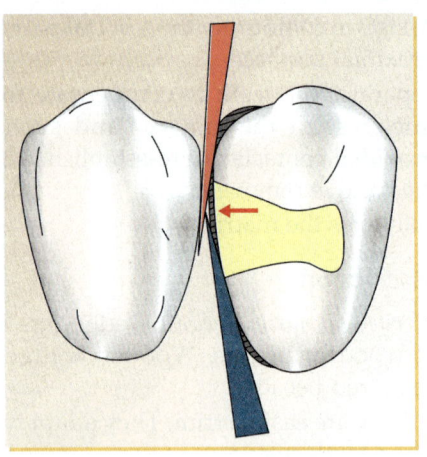

Fig. 4.19c: *Double wedging system: The arrow indicates small space leading to overhanging of restorative material at that area*

lingual embrasure in mandibular posteriors is not practically feasible.

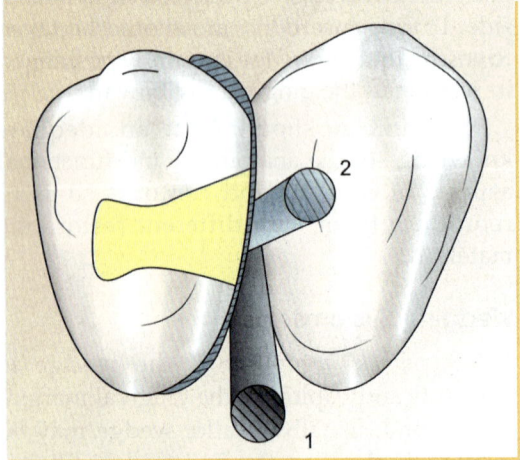

Fig. 4.19b: *Wedge-wedging system: 1. conventional wedge; 2. vertical wedge applied between the matrix band and wedge 1*

one from the lingual embrasure and one from the buccal embrasure (Fig. 4.19c).

However, it has been observed that insertion of wedges from both embrasures leaves some space just below the contact area leading to overhanging of the restorative material at that area. Moreover, insertion of wedges from buccal embrasure in maxillary posteriors and

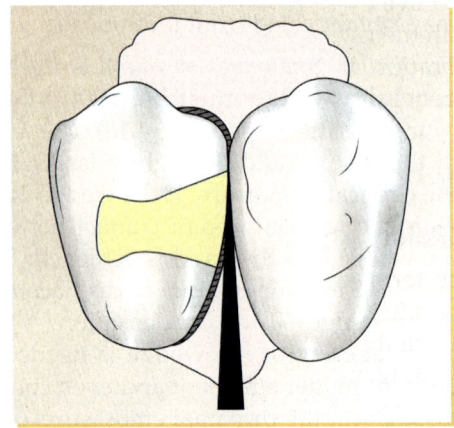

Fig. 4.19d: *Compound supported matrix band*

In such cases, the use of compound supported matrix should be preferred as shown in Fig. 4.19d.

5

Cutting Instruments

In order to perform cavity preparation, the tooth tissues are excised using different instruments. Usually the cavity preparation requires both rotary and hand instruments. Rotary instruments are used for gross reduction whereas hand instruments are effective in producing fine details. And also, with the use of hand instruments, there is no vibration, pain or pressure as compared to rotary instruments. The instruments are:

A. Rotary cutting instruments
B. Hand cutting instruments

A. Rotary Cutting Instruments

The term 'rotary instruments' in dentistry refers to a group of instruments that turn on an axis to perform a work such as cutting, abrading, burnishing, finishing or polishing tooth tissues or a restoration. Majority of dental procedures are accomplished using rotary instruments.

Common Features of Rotary Instruments

The common design features of rotary instruments are (1) shank, (2) neck, and (3) head (Fig. 5.1).

1. *Shank:* The shank is that part of the rotary instrument that fits into the handpiece, accepts the rotary movement from the handpiece and controls the alignment and concentricity of the instrument. The three commonly seen instrument shanks are:
   - Straight

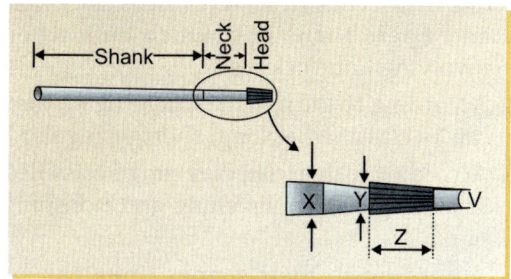

Fig. 5.1: *Parts of rotary cutting instrument. X: Shank diameter, Y: neck diameter, Z: head length and V: taper angle*

   - Latch type
   - Friction grip

2. *Neck:* The neck is the intermediate part of the instrument that connects the shank to the head. It tapers from the shank diameter to a smaller size adjacent to the head. Its size should be so adjusted that it allows maximum visibility and manipulation. Its main function is to transmit rotational and translational forces to the head.

3. *Head:* The head is the working part of the instrument whose cutting edges perform the desired shaping of the tooth structure. The heads of instruments show great variations in design and construction.

Dental Burs

Bur is defined as a rotary cutting instrument with cutting heads of various shapes and two or more sharp edged blades, used as a rotary grinder.

Classification

There are various systems for the classification of burs.

1. According to their mode of attachment to the handpiece, they can be classified as latch type or friction grip type.
2. According to their composition, they can be classified as stainless steel burs, tungsten carbide burs or combination of steel shank and carbide head. The differences of steel and carbide burs are tabulated in Table 5.1.
3. According to their motion, they can be classified as right or left bur. A right bur is one which cuts, when it revolves clockwise and a left bur is one which cuts when revolving anticlockwise.
4. According to the length of their head, they can be classified as long, short or regular.
5. According to their use, they can be classified as cutting burs or finishing and polishing burs.
6. According to their shapes, they can be classified as round, inverted cone, pear shaped, wheel shaped, tapering fissure, straight fissure, end cutting, etc.

Bur Shapes and Sizes

The term 'bur shape' refers to the contour or silhouette of the bur head. The basic head shapes are the round, inverted cone, pear, straight fissure, tapering fissure and end cutting (Fig. 5.2).

a. *Round bur:* A bur with a spherical head is a round bur. It is used for initial tooth preparation, removal of caries, extension of the preparation and for the placement of retentive grooves.

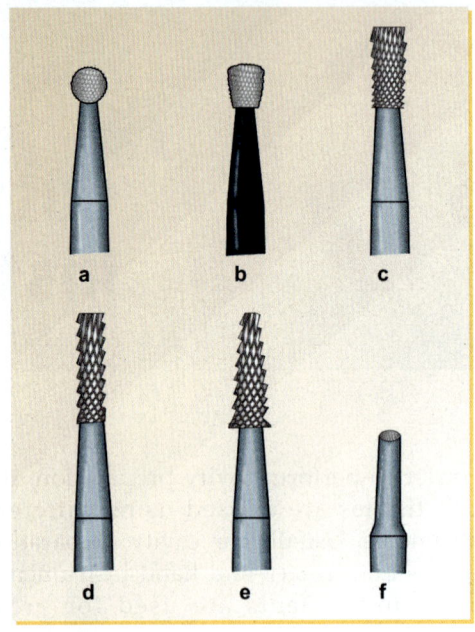

Fig. 5.2a to f: *Bur shapes and sizes*

b. *Inverted cone bur:* The inverted cone bur has a rapidly tapering cone head with sharp angles. The small end of the cone is directed towards the bur shank. It is used for establishing wall angulations and providing undercuts in cavity preparations.

c. *Pear shaped bur:* The pear shaped bur has a slightly tapering cone with rounded angles. The small end of the cone directed towards the bur shank. It is preferably used in occlusal reduction of crown cutting and providing convergence form in amalgam preparations.

d. *Straight fissure bur:* A bur with the head shape of an elongated cylinder. It is used for amalgam cavity preparations.

| Table 5.1: Differences between steel burs and carbide burs | |
Steel burs	*Carbide burs*
• Perform better at low speed	• Perform well at all speeds
• Efficient in cutting enamel only	• Efficient in cutting both enamel and dentin
• Dull rapidly at higher speeds	• Being harder, do not dull rapidly
• Being less brittle than carbide burs, tend to bend causing increase in vibration of the bur	• Being more brittle, tend to fracture when subjected to sudden blow

e. *Tapering fissure bur:* A bur with a tapering cone head with the small end of the cone directed away from the bur shank. It is used for inlay and crown preparations.

f. *End cutting bur:* This bur is cylindrical in shape, with just the end carrying the blades. It is used for carrying the preparation apically without axial reduction.

The size of the bur varies depending upon the need. There is no hard and fast rule for the numbering; however for convenience number 1, 2 and so on is given which signifies the diameter at the tip (Table 5.2).

The minor modifications of the burs include:

• Use of crosscuts
• Extended heads on fissure burs
• Rounding of the sharp tip angles.

Design of a Dental Bur

The actual cutting action of a bur takes place at the edge of the blade present on the bur head. The bur head consists of uniformly spaced blades with depressed areas in between them (Fig. 5.3). These depressed areas are called as the flute or the chip spaces. The number of blades on a bur is usually even. The blades on a cutting bur are usually 6 to 8 to 10 and those on a finishing bur are usually 12 to 40. The greater the number of blades, smoother is the cutting action at low speeds. At high speeds, no more than one blade cuts effectively at any one time.

Blade: The projection on the bur head is known as the blade or the tooth. This terminates in the cutting edge. It has two surfaces: the blade face/rake face and the

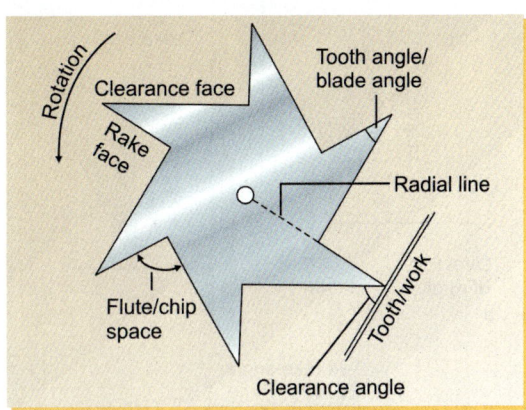

Fig. 5.3: *Cross-section of a bur*

blade back/flank/clearance face. Rake face is the surface of bur blade on the leading edge and clearance face is the surface of the bur blade on the trailing edge.

Rake angle: The rake angle is the most important design characteristic of a bur blade. It is the angle between the rake face and the radial line (line connecting the centre of the bur and the blade). Accordingly, it can be a positive, negative or a zero rake angle (Fig. 5.4).

Land: The plane surface immediately following the cutting edge is called the land.

Clearance angle: The angle between the clearance face and the work (e.g. tooth) is called the clearance angle. If a land is present on the bur, the clearance angle is divided into two: primary clearance angle, i.e. the angle between the land and the work and secondary clearance angle, i.e. the angle between the clearance face and the work. If the clearance face is curved, then it is known as the radial clearance.

Table 5.2: *Commonly used carbide bur: Sizes, shapes and uses*

Bur no./Size (mm)	Shape	Indication of use
¼ (0.40)	Round	Initial entry for cavity preparation, preparation of locks
½ (0.60)	Round	Initial entry for cavity preparations, preparation of locks
2 (1.00)	Round	Excavation at low speed
4 (1.40)	Round	Excavation at low speed
33½ (0.60)	Inverted cone	Undercuts
169 (0.90)	Tapered fissure	Refining inlay preparation, preparation of grooves
330 (0.80)	Pear	Convergence form
245 (0.80)	Pear (long length)	Class II proximal box preparation
271 (1.20)	Tapered fissure	Inlay preparation

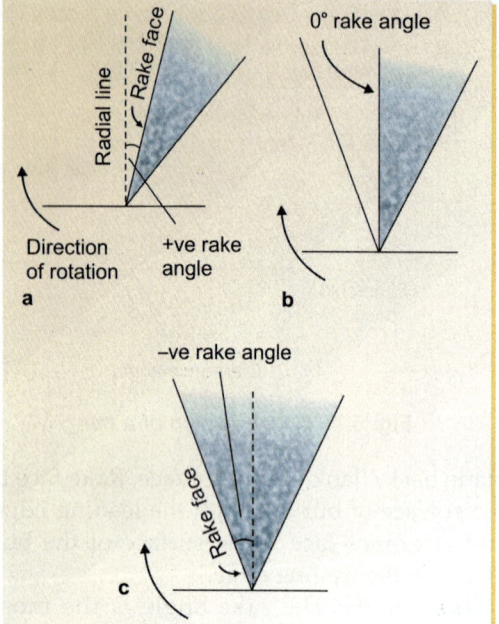

Fig. 5.4: *Rake angles: (a) Positive, (b) radial (zero), (c) negative*

Blade angle/tooth angle: It is the angle between the rake face and the clearance face. In case a land is present, it is the angle between the rake face and the land.

Factors influencing the cutting effectiveness and efficiency of a bur

Cutting effectiveness is the rate of removal of tooth structure in mm/mm or mg/sec; whereas cutting efficiency is the percentage of energy which produces cutting. Cutting efficiency is decreased when some amount of energy is wasted as heat or noise.

The various factors which govern the cutting effectiveness and efficiency are:

- The more positive the rake angle, the greater is the cutting efficiency of the bur.

- As the head of the bur increases in length and diameter, the cutting effectiveness is increased. The movement exerted by the lateral forces also increases so the neck needs to be wider.

- Crosscuts (notches in blade edges) increase the cutting effectiveness at low and medium speeds.

- Symmetrical bur head along with few runouts (displacement of bur head from its axis of rotation) increases effectiveness.

- At a given load, the rate of cutting increases with the rotational speed but not in direct proportion.

- Limited number of teeth/blade increases cutting efficiency; however wear is more and the cutting life is reduced.

Abrasive Instruments

Abrasive instruments constitute the second major category of rotary cutting instruments. The head of these instruments consists of small angular particles of a hard substance held in a matrix of softer material. This softer matrix that holds the particles together is also called the binder. Different materials used as binder are ceramic, metal, rubber, shellac, etc. Rubber and shellac wear away easily and hence are used for delicate abrasion like finishing and polishing.

Abrasive instruments can be grouped into diamond abrasives and other abrasives. Diamond instruments have great clinical impact in operative dentistry because of their long life and great effectiveness in cutting enamel and dentin and hence shall be discussed in detail. Other abrasive instruments include use of silicon carbide, boron carbide, aluminium oxide, garnet and sand for producing grinding wheels, discs or stones, etc.

Diamond Abrasive Instruments

Diamond instruments are preferred over tungsten carbide burs because of their greater resistance to abrasion, lower heat generation and longer life. These instruments consist of three parts: a metal blank, powdered diamond abrasive and a bonding material (Fig. 5.5).

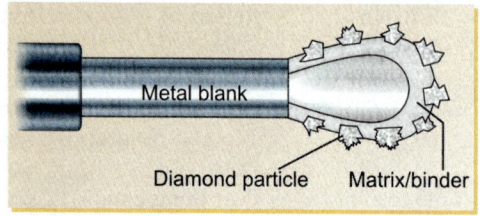

Fig. 5.5: *Diamond instrument (diagrammatic)*

The metal blank resembles a bur without blades. Like any other rotary instrument, it has the same three essential parts: head, neck and shank.

Classification

The various classification systems employed for the burs also hold true for the diamond abrasive instruments. In addition, the latter may also be classified on the basis of the average particle sizes of the abrasive, i.e.

- Coarse grit diamond burs (125–150 µ particle size)
- Medium grit diamond burs (88–125 µ particle size)
- Fine grit diamond burs (60–74 µ particle size)
- Very fine grit diamond burs (38–44 µ particle size)

Head Shapes and Sizes

Diamond instruments are available in a variety of shapes and sizes that correspond to the burs except for the smallest burs.

Due to the lack of any standard and uniform nomenclature for diamond instruments, it becomes necessary to select them visually to obtain the desired shape and size (Fig. 5.6).

Factors influencing the abrasive efficiency and effectiveness.

The clinical performance of diamond abrasive instruments depends upon the following factors:

1. *Size of the abrasive particles:* The larger the size of the particles, deeper is the penetration on the surface of the work; hence rapid removal of material occurs with coarse grit burs compared to medium or fine grit burs.

2. *Shape of the abrasive particles:* The abrasive particles should be irregular in shape for greater efficiency. Irregular particles because of their edges perform better.

3. *Density of the abrasive particles:* Density refers to the number of abrasive particles per unit area. In instruments with high density the particles are closely spaced whereas in those with low density the particles are widely spaced. The effectiveness increases proportionally with the density.

4. *Hardness of the abrasive particles:* For the bur to be efficient, the hardness of the abrasive particle should be greater than the hardness of the work on which it is to be used.

5. *Clogging of the abrasive surface:* Clogging of the abrasive surfaces by grinding debris effects grinding because this partially blocks the penetration of the abrasive particles into the surface. Use of coolants during grinding may wash away the debris and prevent clogging. Hence cleaning is always recommended after each use of bur.

6. *Speed and pressure:* Proper speed and pressure are the major factors determining the life of a bur. The usual cause of failure of abrasive instruments is when excessive pressure is applied on them to increase their cutting rate at inadequate speeds.

7. *Miscellaneous:* These include many uncontrolled operating parameters like individual dental techniques, differences in dental hard tissues, rotation speed, turbine air pressure, differences in handpieces, etc.

Other Abrasive Instruments

Many types of abrasive instruments other than diamonds are used in dentistry. They are used for shaping, finishing and polishing.

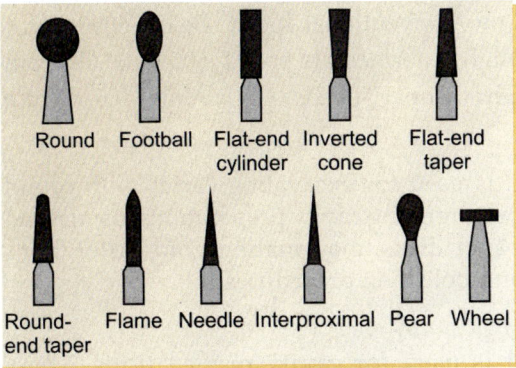

Round   Football   Flat-end cylinder   Inverted cone   Flat-end taper

Round-end taper   Flame   Needle   Interproximal   Pear   Wheel

Fig. 5.6: *Head shapes and sizes of bur*

They can be of two types:
a. Moulded abrasives
b. Coated abrasives

Moulded abrasive instruments have heads manufactured by moulding or pressing a uniform mixture of abrasive and matrix around the roughened end of the shank. The abrasive is distributed throughout the matrix such that new particles are exposed by continual wear. Rigid moulded instruments are used for grinding and sharpening procedures whereas soft moulded instruments are used for finishing and polishing procedures.

Coated abrasive instruments are mostly discs which have a thin layer of abrasive cemented to a flexible backing. This allows the instrument to conform to the surface contour of a tooth or restoration. Unlike the moulded instruments, coated abrasives have to be discarded once they wear off. They are usually used for finishing of restorations (Fig. 5.7a and b).

Types of Handpieces

A handpiece is a device for holding rotating instruments, transmitting power to them and for positioning them intraorally.

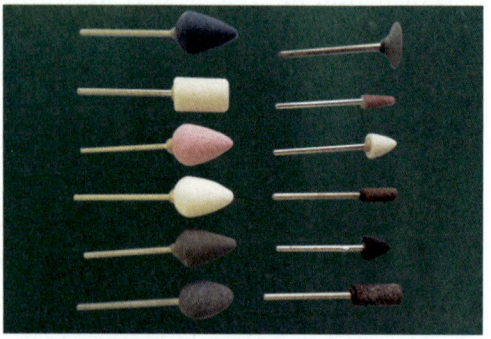

Fig. 5.7a: *Moulded abrasives*

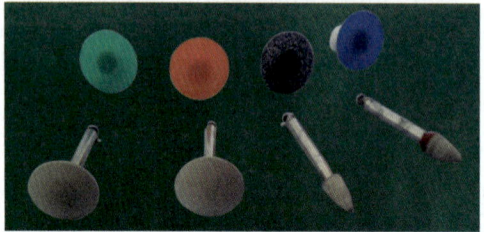

Fig. 5.7b: *Coated abrasives*

Various types of handpieces are available with different technology and speed. These are:

Gear Driven Handpiece

The conventional gear driven handpieces are designed to operate at speeds under 5000 rpm. By the use of several increasing transmissions it is possible to obtain speeds of 100,000 rpm with a gear driven technique.

Proper maintenance is of utmost importance to prevent excessive heat, vibrations and wear within the handpiece.

Water Driven Handpiece

The commercial model is called turbo-jet. It can operate at speeds up to100,000 rpm. The turbo-jet is designed as a compact mobile unit and only electricity is needed to operate it. The handpiece is extremely quiet and efficient.

Belt Driven Handpiece

A belt driven angle handpiece is commercially called the Page-Chayes. All gears were eliminated by having a small belt run inside the handpiece sheath over ball bearing pulleys in the angle sections.

Air Driven Handpiece

The air driven turbine handpiece can run at a speed of approximately 300,000 rpm. The rotary instrument's 1/6 inch shank is held by friction grip. The speed can be regulated depending upon the work load.

Speed Ranges and Uses

Low/conventional speed : Below 6000 rpm
High/intermediate speed : 6000–100,000 rpm
Ultra/super speeds   : Above 100,000 rpm

Low speed

It is used for excavating caries with round burs, refining cavity preparations, using sand paper disks, marginating gold restorations and polishing procedures.

High speed

It is used for cavity preparations. Many procedures such as the placement of retentive grooves and bevels are best performed at high speeds. This speed range is preferred where vision is poor or a more positive sense of touch is needed.

Ultra speed

The ultra speed is desirable for operations as bulk reduction and removing metal restorations. Some cavity preparations may be completed entirely at ultra speeds, lower speed is used for finishing touches.

B. Hand Cutting Instruments

There are various types of hand cutting instruments. However, the basic design is the same.

A hand instrument consists of the following parts (Fig. 5.8):

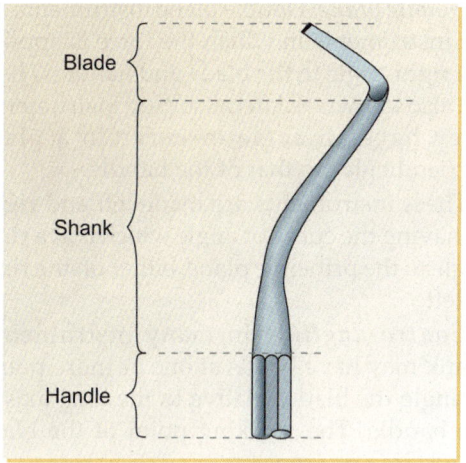

Fig. 5.8: *Parts of hand instrument*

Handle or shaft: It is mostly straight and octagonal in cross-section, and may be serrated to increase friction for hand gripping.

Most hand instrument handles are a continuation of the shank. If the shank and blade are separate from the handle and indented to be screwed into it, the instrument is known as a cone-socket instrument. The handles are available in various sizes and shapes.

Shank: It connects the shaft with the blade. It usually tapers from its connection with the shaft to where the blade begins. Any angulations in the instrument can be placed at the junction of shaft and shank.

Blade/Nib: The working end of cutting instrument is called the blade whereas working end of the non-cutting instrument such as condenser is called a nib (Fig. 5.9). The working surface is called a face. It begins at the angle where the shank is terminated.

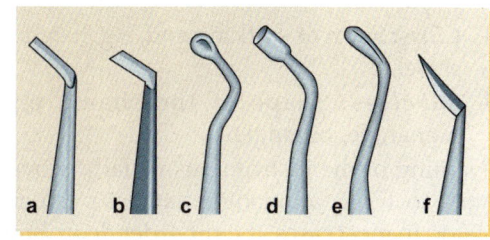

Fig. 5.9: *Characteristics of blade: (a) Hatchet, (b) hoe, (c) excavator, (d) condenser, (e) plastic instrument and (f) carver*

Cutting edge: It is the working part of the instrument. It is usually in the form of a bevel with different shapes.

Blade angle: It is defined as the angle between the long axis of the blade and the long axis of the shaft.

Cutting edge angle: It is defined as an angle between the margins of the cutting edge and the long axis of the shaft (Fig. 5.10).

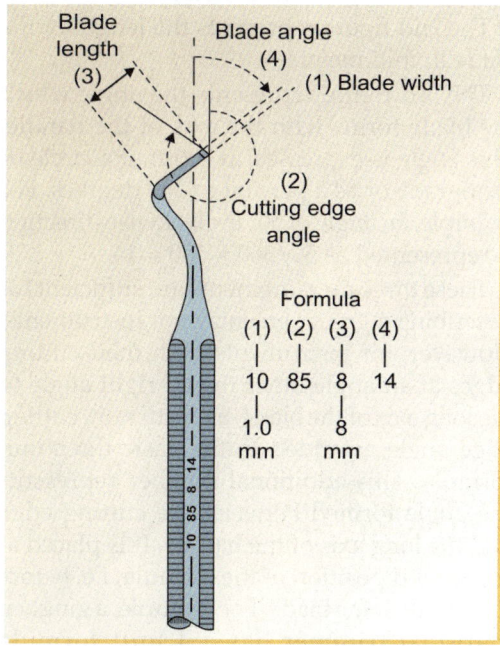

Fig. 5.10: *Instrument formula*

Dr GV Black established a nomenclature for hand instruments, similar to the biological classification.

1. *Order:* Purpose of instrument, e.g. excavator or scaler.
2. *Suborder:* Position or manner of use, e.g. push, pull.
3. *Class:* Form of working end, e.g. hatchet, chisel.
4. *Subclass:* Shape of the shank, e.g. monangle, binangle.

Naming of the instruments usually moves from 4 to 1, e.g. a binangle hatchet push excavator. In most cases, the suborder describing the position or manner of use is variable and non-specific; and for practical purpose it is usually omitted.

Instrument Formula

Dr GV Black gave an instrument formula that describes the dimension and angulations of the hand instruments.

The basic formula consists of three units whose measurements are based upon the metric system.

The 1st figure represents the width of the blade in tenths of a millimeter.

The 2nd figure represents the length of the blade in millimeters.

The 3rd figure represents the angle which the blade forms with the axis of the handle. This angle is expressed in 100th of a circle or centigrade or as a percent of 360 degrees. For example, an angle of 50° in clockwise direction is represented as $50/360 \times 100 = 14$.

These three measurements are sufficient for describing a great percentage of instruments. However, for instruments with their cutting edges at an angle other than a right angle to the long axis of the blade, a fourth unit, cutting edge angle, is added to the basic three-unit formula. This additional number represents the angle formed between the cutting edge and the long axis of the handle. It is placed at the second position of the formula, i.e. before the length of the blade. For example, a gingival marginal trimmer has a 4 unit formula (12½ – 100 – 7 – 14) (Fig. 5.10).

Instrument Design

The main principle of cutting with hand instruments is to concentrate forces on a very thin cross-section of the instruments at the cutting edge. Thus the thinner this cross-section, the more the pressure that is concentrated and the more efficient instrument will be.

Single and Double Plane Instruments

Single plane: Single plane instruments are those in which the force is applied in the same plane as that of the blade and handle. It is also known as direct cutting instruments (Fig. 5.11).

These instruments are made either left or right by placing a bevel on one side of the blade (Fig. 5.12).

Double plane: Double plane instruments are the instruments in which the force is applied at a right angle to the blade and handle. These are also known as lateral cutting instruments. They have an angle or curve in a plane perpendicular to that of the handle.

These instruments are made left and right, by having the curve or angle which is at a right angle to the principle plane, either on the right or left.

Contra-angling: In many instruments, shank may have bends at one or more points to angle the blade relative to the long axis of the handle. The working point of the blade

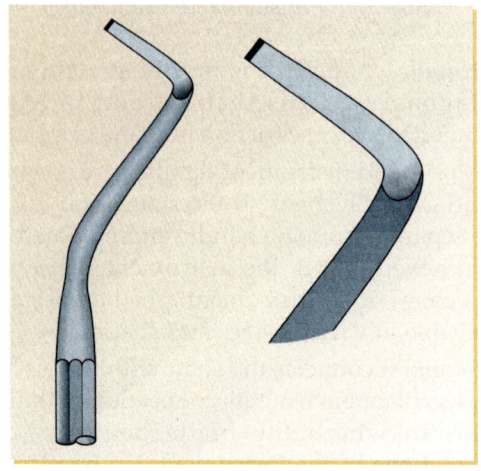

Fig. 5.11: *Single plane instrument (chisel)*

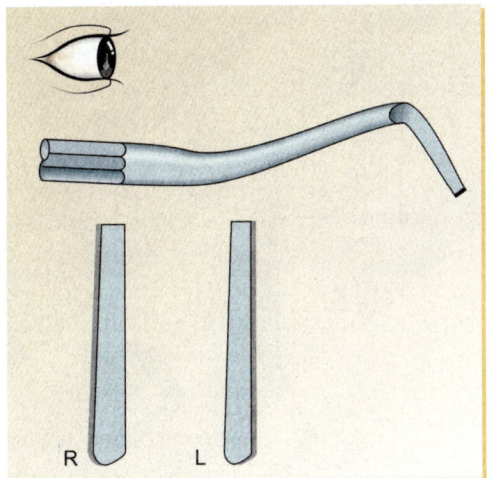

Fig. 5.12: *Hold the instrument with primary cutting edge pointing down and away to determine bevel right (R) and left(L)*

should be placed within 3.0 mm from the axis of the handle. To achieve this, the shank is given certain angulations. This principle is called contra-angling. The contra-angling provides better access and a clear view of the operating field as well as balance the applied forces.

Beveling of Instruments

Single beveled instruments: Most instruments have a single bevel on the cutting edge.

Bi-beveled instruments: Instruments which have two bevels on the opposing side of the instrument blade which meet together to form the cutting edge are called bi-beveled instruments, e.g. ordinary hatchet.

Triple-beveled instruments: Beveling the blade laterally, together with the end, forms three distinct cutting edges in an instrument, e.g. angle former.

Circumferentially beveled instruments: These are usually double-planed instruments where the blade is beveled at all peripheries, e.g. spoon excavator.

Right or left bevel: If the bevel is on the right side of the instrument blade, it is a right sided instrument and if the bevel is on the left side, it is left sided instrument.

Mesially or Distally beveled: When cutting edge is perpendicular to the long axis of handle,

the bevel is not considered right or left but mesial or distal. When the bevel is on the side away from the shaft, the instrument is said to be distally beveled. If bevel is on the side of blade toward the shaft, it is mesially beveled.

Single-ended and double-ended instruments: Single-ended instruments are confined to only one specific function; while double-ended instrument incorporates the right and left or mesial and distal forms of the instrument in the same handle.

When these types of instruments have no angle in the shank or an angle of 12.5° or less, they are used in push (direct cutting) and scraping motions. If this angle in the shank exceeds 12.5°, the instruments could be used in pull (distally beveled) and push (mesially beveled) motions.

Classification

A. Chisels

  a. Straight
  b. Monangle
  c. Binangle
  d. Triple angle

B. Excavators

  a. Hoe
  b. Spoon
  c. Discoid-cleoid

C. Modified form of chisels

  a. Enamel Hatchet
  b. Gingival margin trimmer
  c. Angle former
  d. Wedelstaedt chisel

D. Miscellaneous

  a. Dental probes
  b. Knives
  c. Dental files

A. Chisels

The chisels are used for planing and cleaving. These are characterized by a blade that terminates in a cutting edge formed by a one-sided bevel. Cutting edge of a chisel is at right angle to the shaft (Fig. 5.13).

The chisels are of following types:

a. *Straight chisel:* These have a straight blade in line with the handle and shank. The cutting edge is on one side only (Fig. 5.13a).

b. *Monangle chisels:* In these, the blade is placed at an angle to the shaft. It may be mesially (Standard) or distally (reverse) beveled (Fig. 5.13b).

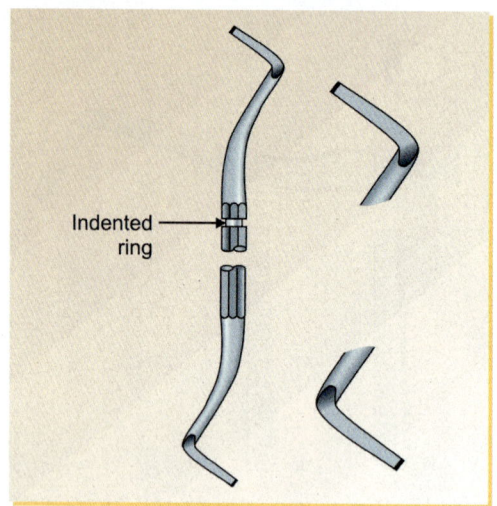

Fig. 5.14: *Binangle chisel (arrow showing indented ring)*

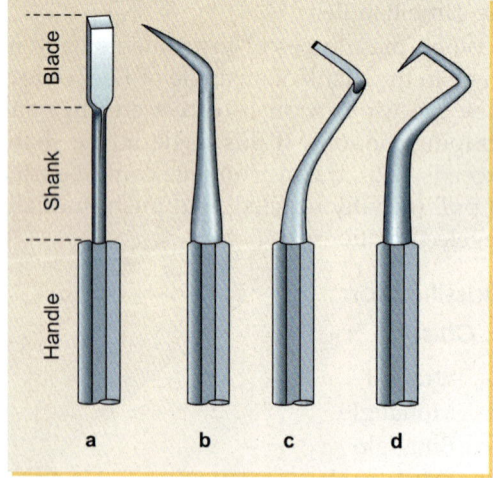

Fig. 5.13: *Chisels. (a) Straight, (b) monangle, (c) binangle and (d) triple angled*

c. *Binangle chisels:* These have two angles between the shaft and the blade. It may be mesially or distally beveled (Figs 5.13c and 5.14).

d. *Triple-angle chisels:* These have three angles in the shank and are usually used to flatten pulpal floor. It may also be mesially or distally beveled (Fig. 5.13d).

B. Excavators

Excavators are used for excavation and removal of caries and sharpening or refinement of the internal parts of the cavity preparation (Fig. 5.15).

The excavators are of following types:

a. *Hoe:* It is a form of chisel in which the angle of the blade is more than 12.5 and may approach a right angle, i.e. 25 centigrade. It is a single-planed instrument, which can be

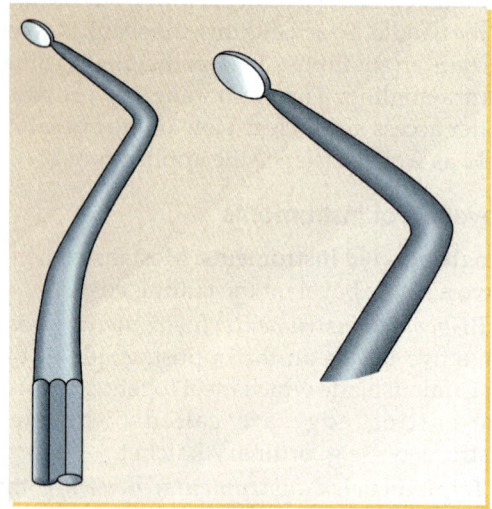

Fig. 5.15: *Spoon excavators*

mesially or distally beveled and used with pull motion.

Hoe is used for cutting mesial and distal walls of premolars and molars.

b. *Spoon:* In these instruments, the cutting edge is ground to a semicircular circumferential bevel and sharpened to a thin edge. These are available in pairs with the blade of one curved to the right, and the blade of the other curved to the left. The spoon excavators are double-planed instruments with right or left cutting movement only.

The spoon excavators are used for removal of decayed dentin.

c. *Discoid-Cleoid (claw-like):* It is similar to the spoon excavator, except that the blade resembles a claw, hence the name 'cleoid'.

Earlier it was used to excavate caries from difficult areas; however, presently it is used to carve the occlusal surface of amalgam restoration.

C. Modified form of Chisels

a. *Enamel hatchet:* Any instrument where the cutting edge, is parallel or near parallel to the plane of instruments is called a hatchet. If the blade of a hatchet is at perpendicular angles to the shaft, the cutting edge would be parallel to the shaft.

These are paired, i.e. right and left hatchets, with an indented ring on the shank or shaft of the right instrument of the pair as identification mark. These are used for cleaving and planing enamel and dentin.

Uses: Rounding or beveling of axiopulpal line angle and beveling gingival enamel margins of proximocclusal proportions.

b. *Gingival margin trimmer (GMT):* It is a modified form of hatchet. Two distinct modifications of the basic hatchet design are:

  i. Cutting edge of a hatchet is at a perpendicular angle to the axis of the blade while cutting edge of a gingival margin trimmer is at an angle other than a perpendicular angle to the axis of the blade (so a 4-unit formula).

  ii. Hatchet has a straight blade (single plane); the blade of a GMT is curved (Double plane). It is paired with right and left bevels (Fig. 5.16).

c. *Angle former:* It is a modified form of chisel. In this instrument, the primary cutting edge is sharpened at an angle (usually 80–85 degrees) to the axis of the blade. Blade of the angle former is beveled on both the

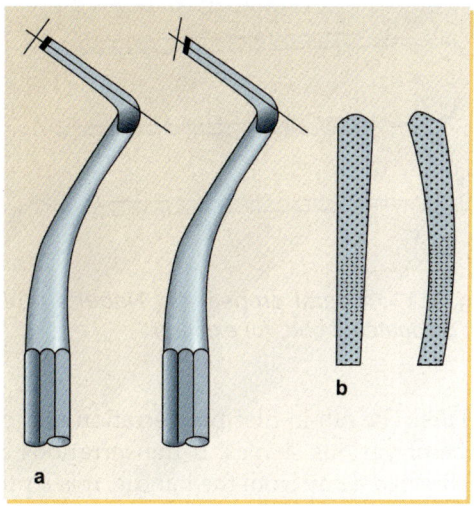

Fig. 5.16: *Enamel hatchet (a), compared with gingival marginal trimmer (b)*

sides, to form three cutting edges. The acute cutting angle being directed to the right or left makes the angle former a paired instrument. Right of the pair is identified by an indented ring.

It is used to accentuate line and point angles in the internal outline form. It is frequently used in cavity preparation for cohesive gold to establish retention form.

d. Wedelstaedt chisel: It is like a straight chisel, but with a slight vertical curvature in its shank. It is beveled on one side only which can be placed mesially or distally.

D. Miscellaneous

a. *Dental probes:* Various types of probes are available, which can be straight, curved or graduated (used in periodontology) (Fig. 5.17).

b. *Knives:* Nibs of these instruments carry knife-edged faces on one of their sides only. The commonly used knives are finishing knives, amalgam knives and gold knives. They are used for trimming off excess filling material on the gingival, facial or lingual margins of a proximal restoration or trimming and contouring the surface of a class V restoration.

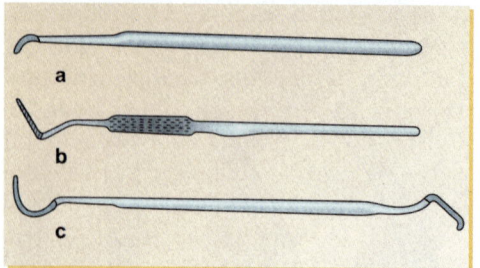

Fig. 5.17: *Dental probes. (a) Naber's probe, (b) graduated probe, (c) explorer*

c. *Files:* The nib in files has serration and can be of various shapes. If the serrations are directed away from the handle, it is a push file and the serrations are directed towards the handle, it is a pull file.

These are used for smoothening of cavo-surface margins.

Methods of Use

- The instruments are used from the bevel side.
- Use the instruments parallel to the walls, while working occluso-gingivally; hold the instrument 90 degree to the walls while working proximoaxially.
- The blade of the instrument is kept at 90 degrees to the cavosurface margin.

Basically there are four grasps used with hand instruments, which are as follows:

1. *Pen grasp:* It is similar to the method of holding a pen. The 1st and 2nd fingers contact the instrument, while the tip of 3rd and 4th fingers are placed on the adjoining teeth (as rests).

   The position of 2nd finger is important for good control and thrust to the instrument. This way, due to greater length of the 2nd finger, the application point for the force will be near the working point of the instrument.

2. *Inverted pen grasp:* This is similar to the pen grasp, but the hand is rotated so that the palm is facing upwards. It is usually used in upper teeth.

3. *Palm and thumb grasp:* It is similar to the method of holding a knife. The handle is placed in the palm of the hand and grasped by the four fingers, while the thumb rests on an area other than that being operated on. A supporting rest provided by the thumb is necessary because digital control is somewhat insufficient.

   It may be useful on maxillary teeth particularly the right side, when working from the right rear chair position.

4. *Modified palm and thumb grasp:* When it is feasible to rest the thumb on the same tooth being operated or on a tooth immediately adjacent, the modified palm and thumb grasp may be used.

   The handle of the instrument is held between the pulps of the thumb and the 1st and 2nd fingers. The 3rd and 4th fingers are about half closed; they contact the handle under the 1st joint of each finger and press the handle against the distal area of the palm.

   Rests: Rests are used to stabilize the hand during operating procedures and these also act as guards when force is applied.

   Whenever feasible, the rest should be on the arch being operated on and preferably on the same quadrant.

   Guards: Guards are finger positions of the hand opposite the one using the instrument, to steady the parts being operated on and to protect them from injury in case the instrument accidentally slips off the working surface.

   These should be used particularly when adjacent teeth are not available as rests or when rests should be obtained on soft tissues or on the opposite arch.

Advantages of Hand Cutting Instruments

- They are self limited in cutting enamel, i.e. they will not cut sound enamel, but cut only enamel undermined by loss of dentin.
- They can remove large pieces of under-mined enamel quickly, thus saving time and effort.

- No vibration or heat accompanies the cutting, making it painless and with no adverse effects on the tooth tissues.
- Most efficient means of precise cutting, especially when cutting is needed adjacent to important anatomy.
- Create smoothest surface of all cutting instruments.
- Have the longest life span, as can be re-sharpened.

Hand cutting instruments provide a better control on cutting and are more compliant to patients. Though their use is declining now-a-days due to advent of rotary cutting instruments, their advantages and precision cannot be overlooked.

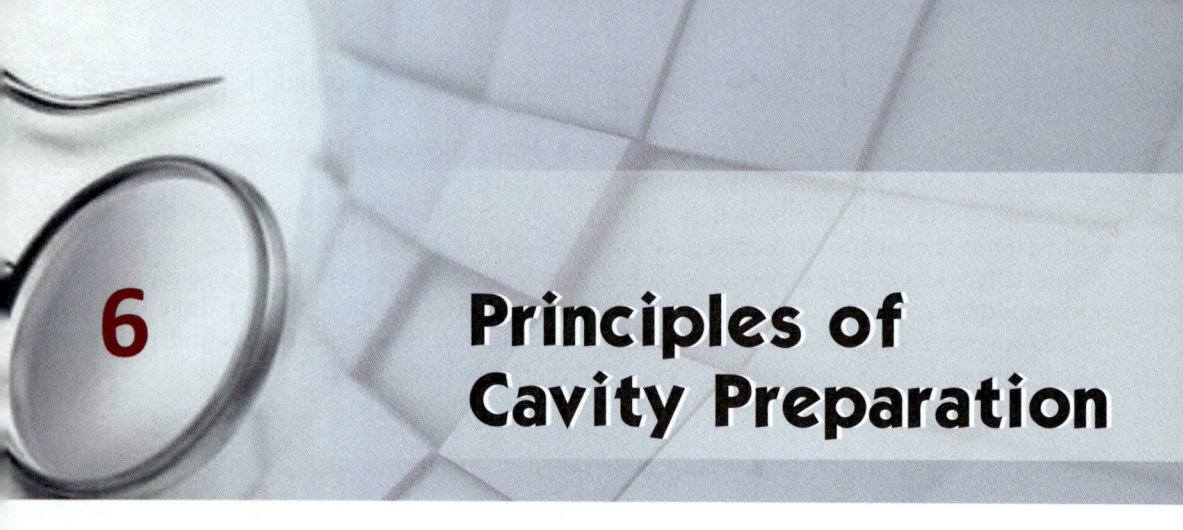

6

Principles of Cavity Preparation

The preparation of a cavity should be carried out in an orderly sequence, following certain principles. Dr GV Black suggested six principles for cavity preparation, which by and large are followed, though each principle has been modified keeping in view the advancement in restorative materials. The cavity preparation is accomplished through systematic procedures based on these principles. Thorough knowledge of tooth anatomy viz. direction of enamel rods, thickness of enamel at various places, size and position of the pulp and the relation of the crown with the gingival tissue is mandatory. These principles are as follows:

1. Outline form
2. Resistance and retention forms
3. Convenience form
4. Removal of remaining carious dentin
5. Finishing of the enamel walls and margins
6. Toilet of the cavity

1. Outline Form

Dr GV Black, described outline form as *the area of tooth surface or the enamel margin to be included in the finished cavity.*

This is basically the external outline form. The internal outline form, however, includes the inner dimensions and details of the prepared cavity. In young teeth, the internal outline form should be prepared carefully as pulp chamber is large and more superficial.

Following factors influence the outline form:
a. Extent of the carious lesion
b. The proximity of the lesion to other defects in the enamel
c. The relationship of adjacent and opposing teeth
d. The relationship of soft tissue
e. Esthetic considerations
f. Type of material to be used

A. Outline form for Occlusal Cavities
(Figs 6.1 and 6.2)

The outline form for occlusal cavities dictates as:

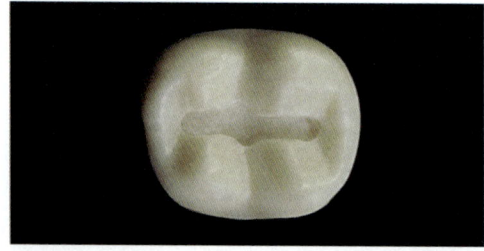

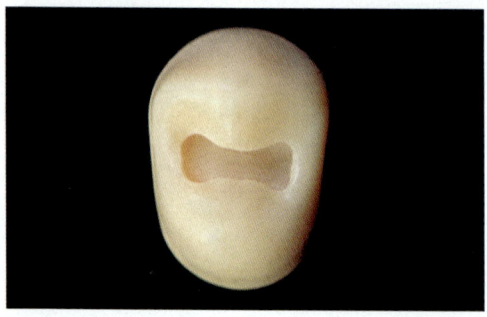

Figs 6.1 and 6.2: *Outline form for occlusal cavities*

a. Extend the cavity margins to sound tooth structure and remove all unsupported enamel.

b. Include all susceptible fissures in the outline form. This phenomenon of 'Extension for Prevention' was first suggested by Marshall Ebb and was later adopted by Black.

c. Two cavities having less than 0.5 mm of sound tooth structure between them should be joined.

d. Cavity margins should not terminate in high stress areas, such as cusp heights or ridge crests.

e. Extend the margins to allow sufficient access for cavity refinement, restoration placement and finishing procedures.

B. Outline form for Proximal Cavities
(Figs 6.4 and 6.5)

The outline form for proximal cavities dictates as:

- Position and crest of healthy gingiva, age of the patient vis-à-vis the epithelial attachment.
- Dimensions of contact area to be restored
- Extent of caries at and around the contact area
- Oral hygiene of the patient
- Possible forces of mastication
- Placement of margins (Fig. 6.3)

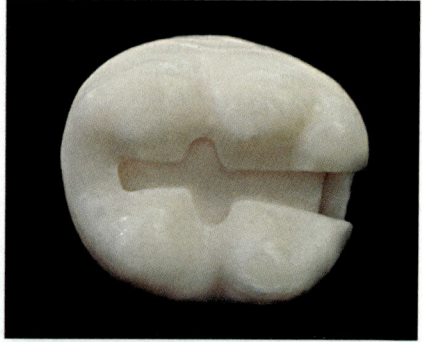

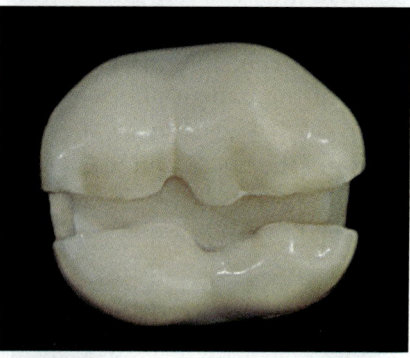

Figs 6.4 and 6.5: *Outline form for proximal cavities*

There are no set rules in cavity preparation that cannot be modified; however, these modifications should be within limits so as not to defy the basic principles.

There are certain conditions which may warrant restricted or reduced extension:

- Proximal cavities
- Root proximities
- Esthetic requirements

Certain conditions may require increased extension:

- Mental or physical handicap patients
- Advanced age of the patient
- When additional resistance or retention is required
- Need to adjust tooth contours

The rationale for modifying cavity design reflects the development of new materials, modification of traditional materials with better physical properties, awareness of patients towards better oral health, coupled with the use of fluorides and improved equipment in the dental office. The principle

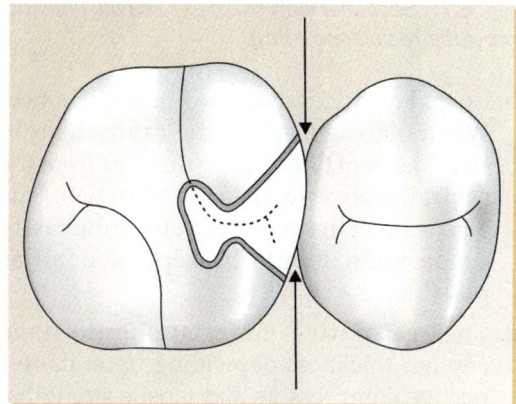

Fig. 6.3: *Axial margins should clear the contact area and extend into embrasures for self cleansing action*

of 'extension for prevention' is being questioned in the light of newer materials and techniques.

C. Outline form for Gingival/Cervical Cavities (Fig. 6.6)

The outline form for the gingival/cervical cavities dictates as:

- In young patients the restoration is covered by gingiva, i.e. most of the restorative margins are kept sub-gingival. However, in older patients, the margins can be kept supra-gingival.
- Abnormal occlusal contacts and eating pattern of the patient affects planning of cervical cavities.
- Contour of the buccal/lingual surfaces
- Extent of the caries
- Oral hygiene of the patient

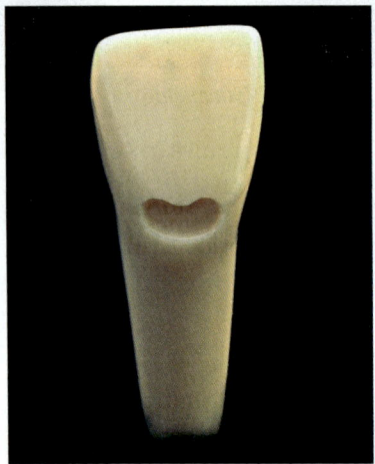

Fig. 6.6: *Outline form for cervical cavities*

D. Outline form for Root Caries

The outline form for root caries is controlled mainly by the site of the lesion, extent of the caries, age of the patient and the oral hygiene. By and large, root caries is managed by excavating the caries and restoring without any injudicious extension.

2. Resistance and Retention Forms

The resistance and retention forms are interrelated and interdependent; that is why they are considered simultaneously. A few

authors have even preferred the term 'retention-resistance form'.

'Resistance form' may be defined as *that shape and configuration of the cavity that best enables both the restoration and the tooth to withstand occlusal forces without fracture.* The resistance form is in direct relation to the degree of exposure of the restoration to the occlusal forces.

There are some fundamental factors, which are to be followed in obtaining resistance form, which are as follows:

a. The cavity should be prepared as a box with a flat floor. Flat floor resists the occlusal stresses, being at right angle to such forces (Fig. 6.7). If necessary the flat seats can be increased. The excavated areas are filled with suitable cements so as to create a flat surface for final restoration (Fig. 6.8a and b).

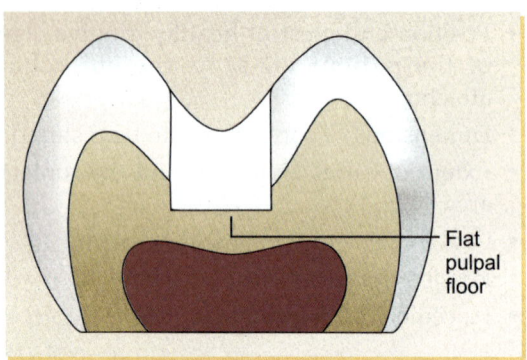

Fig. 6.7: *Sectional view of a class I cavity (flat floor provides resistance form)*

b. Cusps and ridges should not be undermined. When a fissure is cut, the cavity margin should extent to 1/3rd the distance from the central groove to cusp tip (Fig. 6.9). The extension of the external walls of the cavity preparation should be kept as small as possible.

c. The restorative material should have enough thickness depending upon its respective compressive and tensile strengths.

d. Weakened tooth structure should be enveloped or included in cavity form to prevent damage from lateral forces.

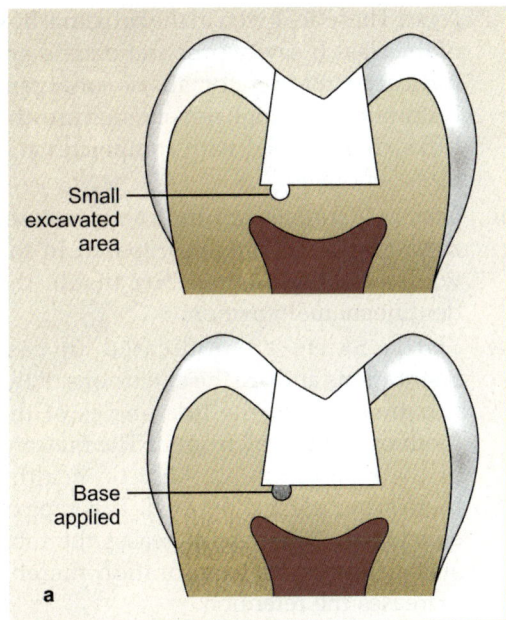

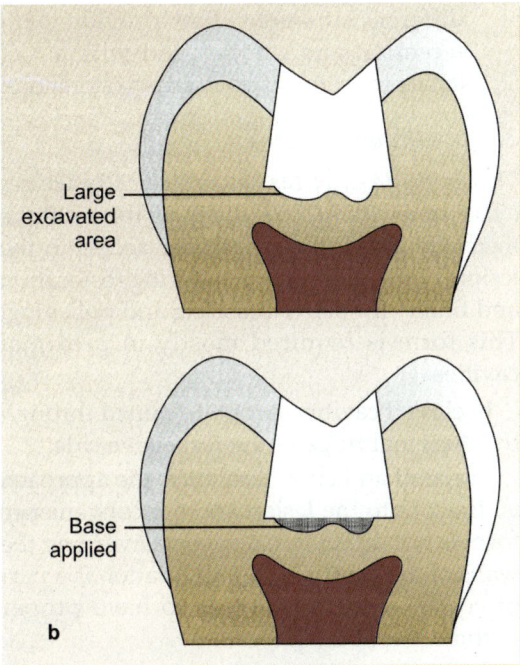

Fig. 6.8: *(a) Small excavated area and application of base of suitable cement, (b) large excavated area and application of base of suitable cement*

e. Roundening of line angles avoids stresses directly on to the tooth, thereby resistance

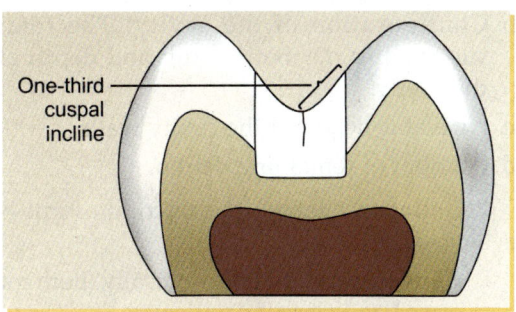

Fig. 6.9: *The cavity margin should extend to one-third the distance from the central groove to the cusp tip*

to fracture is increased. The sharp line angles lead to poor resistance form (Fig. 6.10).

f. The minimal thickness of amalgam and cast gold to resist fracture is approximately 1.5 mm, though little more depth is required for amalgam to achieve the requisite bulk. However, in composites and glass-ionomers, the depth is not the criteria for achieving resistance form.

'Retention form' may be defined as *the shape and configuration of the cavity that enables the restoration to be retained in that cavity under all types of tipping and tilting stresses.*

The retention form usually varies with the type of the material. However, following features should be considered for any restorative material.

a. Magnitude of the occlusal forces and the area of the restoration, which will be under the occlusal load.

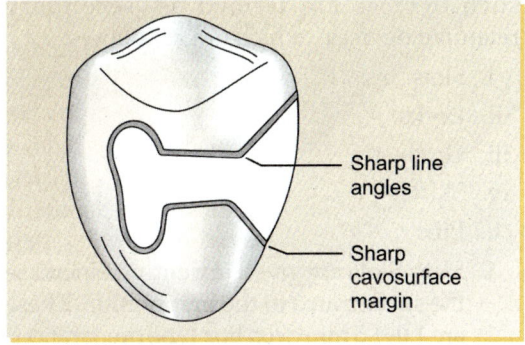

Fig. 6.10: *Sharp line angles lead to poor resistance form at the cavity restoration interface*

b. Configuration of the cavity. The total surface area, i.e. both width and depth of the cavity.

c. Available height of the cavity walls

d. Amount of remaining dentin.

For **silver amalgam**, the retention form is achieved by:

i. Converging the walls occlusally (both for class I and class II cavities)

ii. Marginal ridge is to be conserved

iii. Slight undercuts can be given in the dentin

For **cast restorations** the retention form is achieved by:

i. Parallelism of walls. A slight divergence (2°–5°) can be given for proper withdrawal of the pattern. In case the available height of the walls is less, the divergence should be kept minimum.

ii. Occlusal extension is mandatory even if no occlusal caries is present since it prevents tilting.

iii. Reverse bevel at the gingival wall will prevent tipping movements.

In **composites**, the bonding agents used are helpful in achieving the retention. The surface area of the cavity and the type of bonding agent, both aid in the retention form.

Many a times, the prepared cavity is not retentive even after providing necessary features. In such cases, other devices are used which provide extra retention and even reinforce the tooth in certain conditions. All such devices are termed as 'secondary retentive devices', which are as follows:

i. Slots

ii. Locks

iii. Grooves

iv. Skirts

v. Pins

i. *Slots:* Slots are given in dentin to increase the surface area of the preparation. These are 1.0–1.5 mm deep box type preparations which can be given in occlusal wall or gingival wall or both.

ii. *Locks:* These are given in the proximal box of the class II cavity preparation and are indicated mainly for silver amalgam restorations. Though not of much use, the locks are also tried with composites and glass-ionomers.

iii. *Grooves:* Grooves are indicated for cast restorations. These are prepared in the walls of the proximal box inside the dentinoenamel junction.

iv. *Skirts:* Skirts are indicated in cast restorations and are the extensions of the proximal box at the line angles of the tooth or even away from it. The margins of the restoration are kept on healthy tooth structure and beveled. This type of enveloping the walls increases the total surface area of the restoration thereby increases the retention.

v. *Pins:* Various types of pins are available in different shapes and sizes suitable for different situations. Pins provide extra retention and can be used with silver amalgam, composites and cast restorations.

3. Convenience Form

This is the form of the cavity, which visualizes lesion more clearly. The shape of the cavity is modified so as to have proper access to the lesion, better manipulation during restoration and finally for better finishing and polishing. This form is required mostly in proximal cavities.

In class II cavities, access is gained through the marginal ridge of the respective side.

In class I and class V cavities, the approach is direct onto the lesion and the convenience form is not difficult to achieve. Diverging the walls of the cavity in cast restoration is a part of convenience form so as to have proper withdrawal of the pattern.

4. Removal of Remaining Carious Dentin

Elimination of any infected carious tooth structure or faulty restoration left in the cavity preparation is the fourth principle. After preparing the cavity with adequate width and depth, the remaining portion is checked for any left over caries. The site and location of such caries is important since it will dictate the future modification of the preparation.

In no case soft and infected caries should be left over the pulp. Such residual caries leads to pulpal inflammation and subsequently slow death of pulp.

In case of children and young pulps, the left over caries is best tolerated. And also, vital pulp is needed for proper root formation.

5. Finishing the Enamel Walls and Margins

The cavosurface margins and the enamel at the cavity walls are finished in such a way so that the adaptation of the restorative material is improved.

This procedure provides maximum strength to both the tooth and the restorative material especially at the margins.

Finishing of enamel margins depend upon the following features:

i. Location of the margins vis-à-vis direction of the enamel rods

ii. Type of the restorative material to be used

iii. Degree of smoothness required

iv. Previous restorative material used, if any

Thorough knowledge of anatomy of enamel rods is mandatory for proper finishing.

- The rods extend full length from dentino-enamel junction to outer enamel surface
- The enamel rods radiate from dentino-enamel junction to the external surface of the enamel. In axial sections, occlusally, the rods make a +20° to +30° angle with the long axis of the tooth. In the middle, they are perpendicular and in the gingival third they make an angle of –5° to –10°.
- The rods usually converge towards concave surfaces and diverge towards convex surfaces.

Finishing of enamel margins is carried out almost in every restorative material. In case of silver amalgam, butt end of the cavosurface margins are preferred because of poor edge strength of amalgam. The gingival wall is slightly beveled, thereby removing the unsupported enamel rods. A short bevel is given for cast gold restoration.

6. Toilet of the Cavity

The procedure involves removal of all debris and cut dentinal chips from the walls of the cavity. Warm water can be utilized along with drying with oil free air. Mild acidic solutions have been tried but are not of much use.

The over-drying of the cavity with compressed air, etc. is also avoided, especially in composite restorations; the bonding agents are hydrophilic and prefer wet dentin.

After cleaning the cavity, care should be taken so that saliva or moisture should not enter in the cavity.

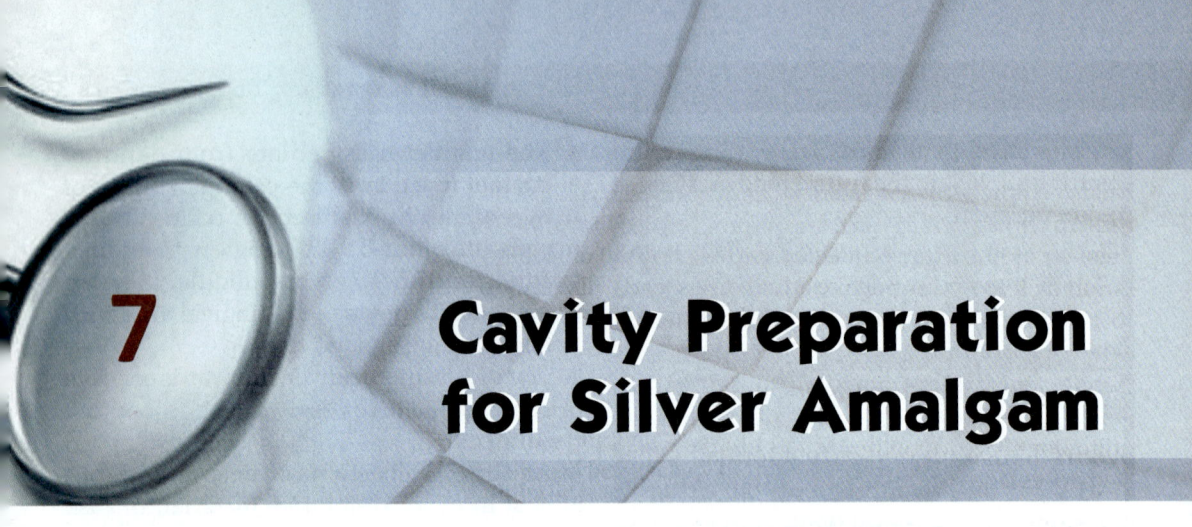

7

Cavity Preparation for Silver Amalgam

Silver amalgam, undoubtedly, is the most commonly and widely used restorative material. The advantages of silver amalgam, especially over esthetic restorative materials have been established. Except for the colour, all other properties are better in silver amalgam.

Silver amalgam if properly manipulated produces a restoration, which could provide many years of service.

The cavity preparation along with manipulation of silver amalgam is important to achieve successful restoration.

Advantages

1. The manipulation viz. mixing, squeezing and condensing, etc. is very simple.
2. It can be given in any class and any size of the cavity.
3. The expansion and contraction falls within permissible range ($\pm$ 0.2 percent).
4. Physical characteristics are comparable to enamel and dentin.
5. Biologically stable
6. Economical
7. Allergic reactions are very rare

Disadvantages

1. Esthetically poor.
2. Low copper or conventional silver amalgams may exhibit degradation and ditching with time.
3. Excessive cavity cutting is required because bulk provides strength.

4. Tensile strength is less.
5. Silver is a good thermal conductor, so base is required under these restorations.

COMPOSITION OF ALLOY

The advantage of alloying metals is that when a new compound is formed, it possesses properties that are not present in single element. Amalgam is the mixture of mercury with one metal or alloy. Mercury, having the property of dissolving other metals, produces a plastic mass.

Conventional silver alloy comprises of the following components:

Silver (Ag)	68–72% (wt %)
Tin (Sn)	25–27%
Copper (Cu)	2–6%
Zinc (Zn)	0–3%

However recently, alloys with copper contents more than 6% and may be up to 30% have been introduced with the idea of eliminating γ_2 phase.

The early alloys were admixed alloy having silver copper eutectic; however, later they were modified to make it single composition.

A. Admixed/Blended Alloy

This single alloy is a mixture of two types of particles viz. lathe cut low copper alloy particles and spherical eutectic (silver copper) alloy particles.

Admixed alloys are of following two types:

i. *Type I alloy:* It contains two parts of conventional lathe cut particles and one part by weight of silver copper eutectic alloy.

ii. *Type II alloy:* It is the reverse of type I alloy, i.e. it contains two parts of spherical silver copper alloy and one part of conventional alloy.

B. Single Composition/All in one Alloy

In this powder, each particle of the alloy has the same chemical composition that is why they are called single composition alloys.

These may be of the following types:

i. *Ternary alloys:* The composition is silver 60%, tin 25%, copper 15%.

ii. *Quaternary alloys:* Silver 60%, copper 13%, tin 24%, indium 3%.

Effect of Constituent Metals on the Properties of Silver Amalgam

Silver

- Increases strength
- Decreases flow
- Increases setting expansion
- Resists tarnish and corrosion
- Reduces setting time by accelerating the setting process
- It whitens the alloy

Tin

- Reduces strength
- It helps in amalgamation since tin has great affinity for mercury

- Increases setting time
- Decreases setting expansion
- Reduces the resistant to tarnish and corrosion

Copper

- Increases strength
- Reduces flow
- Increases setting expansion
- Makes the alloy less susceptible to imperfection during manipulation.

Zinc

- Prevents oxidation during manufacturing of alloy
- Contributes to the cleanliness or workability of silver amalgam during trituration and condensation
- Responsible for delayed expansion if zinc containing alloys are contaminated with water/saliva
- Makes the alloy less susceptible to imperfection during manipulation.

CAVITY PREPARATION

The cavity preparation for silver amalgam envisages all the principles given by GV Black. The individual cavity design and modifications are described.

Class I (Fig. 7.1)

The carious lesions occur mostly in occlusal pits and fissures and also the buccal/lingual pits of posterior teeth and lingual pits of anterior teeth.

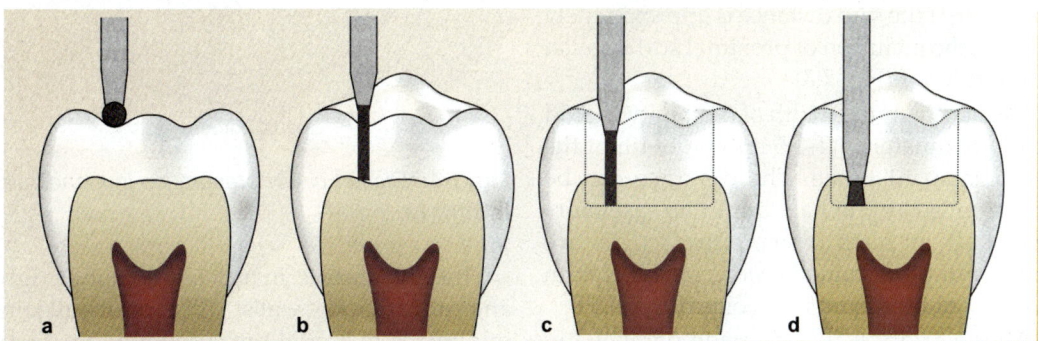

Fig. 7.1a to d: *(a) Deepest or most carious pit is entered with small round bur, (b) No. 1 fissure bur is used for further preparation, (c) No.1 fissure bur 0.5 mm below the DEJ, (d) flat pulpal floor is made with inverted cone bur*

a. Cavities on the occlusal pits and fissures

In case the caries is only on occlusal pits and fissures, the outline is planned. After planning, a small round bur is used to enter the deepest or most carious pit, moving the bur parallel to the long axis of the tooth crown. When the bur touches the dentinoenamel junction or slightly into the dentin, the No.1 fissure bur is used for further preparation. The fissure bur is moved along the fissures maintaining the uniform depth (1.5 mm). The flat pulpal floor is created with facial and lingual walls almost parallel (Fig. 7.2a).

A 10° occlusal divergence at mesial and distal marginal ridges is created. This procedure prevents the undermining of marginal ridges (Fig. 7.2b).

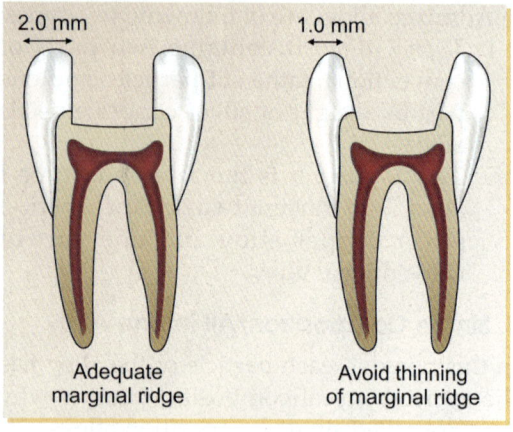

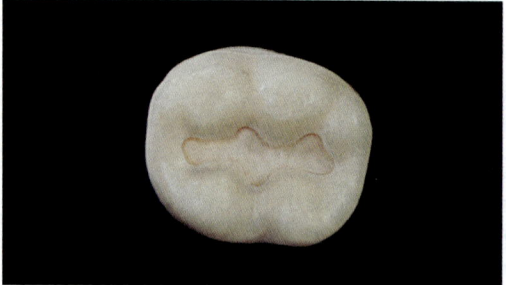

Fig. 7.3: *Extension of cavity outline along marginal ridge*

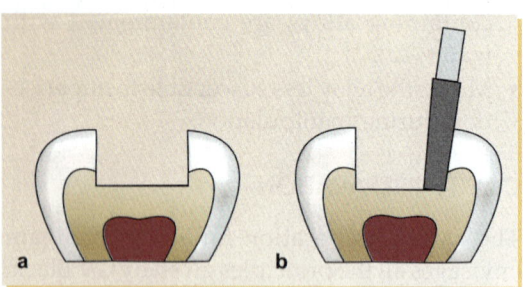

Fig. 7.2a and b: *(a) Flat pulpal floor, (b) mesial and distal walls given 10° divergence*

The distance of margins of such an extension to the proximal surface must not be less than 1.5 mm in premolars and 2.0 mm in molars. In case the distance is slightly less, the divergence of the walls can be avoided. However, if the said distance is approximately 1.0 mm, the inclusion of proximal surfaces can be considered (Fig. 7.3).

The buccolingual width of the cavity should be approximately 1.0–1.5 mm or 1/4th of the intercuspal distance. The distance can be compromised up to half, but in no case more than half. In such cases, either cusps are covered or undermined lesions are filled with glass-ionomer cements or composites.

All the cavity walls are made parallel and perpendicular to each other. These walls should be joined by definite line and point angles, which are kept rounded (Fig. 7.4).

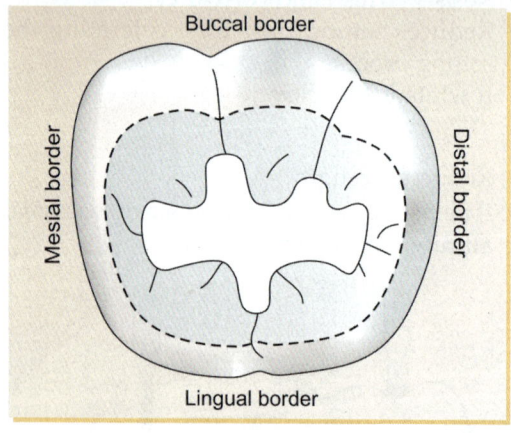

Fig. 7.4: *Class I cavity preparation in mandibular first molar*

The cavosurface margins are kept at right angle to the cavity walls. This type of butt joint minimizes marginal breakdown of amalgam (Bevels not given). The depth of the cavity is placed 0.5 mm below the dentinoenamel junction. This much depth provides bulk of silver amalgam as well as retention because of elasticity of dentin.

The crossing ridges should be preserved as far as possible (transverse ridge and oblique ridge). If the caries involves more than half the planes of these ridges, the total ridge can be involved (Fig. 7.5).

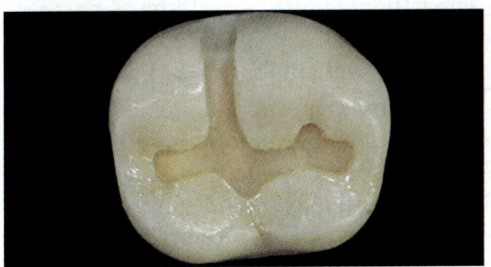

Fig. 7.5: *Class I cavity with buccal complex in mandibular first molar*

Many a time, caries extends at one or more points below the otherwise flat pulpal floor. Such carious lesions are either excavated with fine excavators or removed with small round burs (Fig. 7.6). These depressions in the pulpal floor are filled with sedative cement like zinc oxide eugenol or calcium hydroxide (Fig. 7.7).

b. Cavities on pits and fissures on the occlusal 2/3rd of buccal and lingual surfaces of posterior teeth and lingual pits of anterior teeth

In case where the pits and fissures of only one surface are involved (facial or lingual), it is necessary to remove the decayed portion and widen it accordingly to remove undermined enamel. The shape is generally oblong or triangular (Fig. 7.8). The axial wall is kept flat and the surrounding walls are made slightly convergent towards the cavosurface margins. The cervical wall should follow the contour of cementoenamel junction.

Most commonly, the carious lesions at the buccal and lingual sides are connected to the occlusal lesions. In such cases, the occlusal portion is prepared as described in Class I. Care

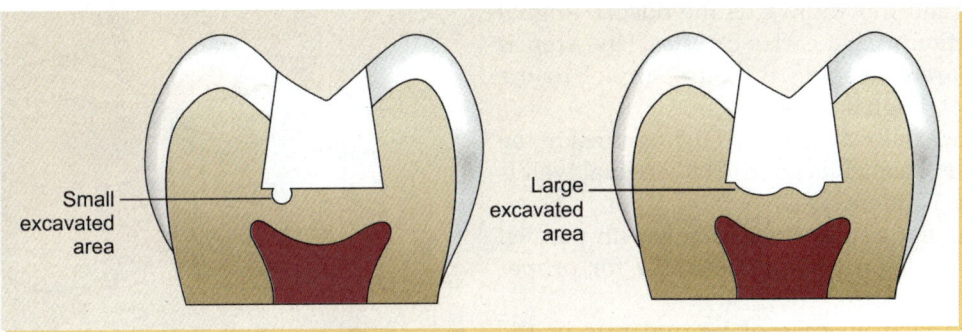

Small excavated area

Large excavated area

Fig. 7.6: *Excavated area*

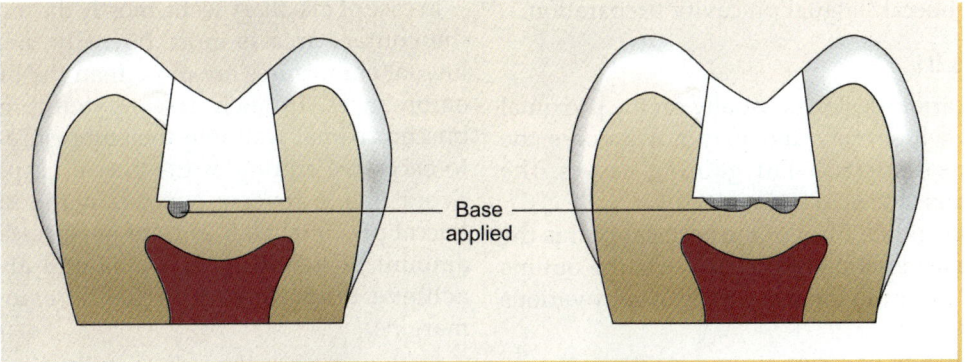

Base applied

Fig. 7.7: *Application of base of suitable cement*

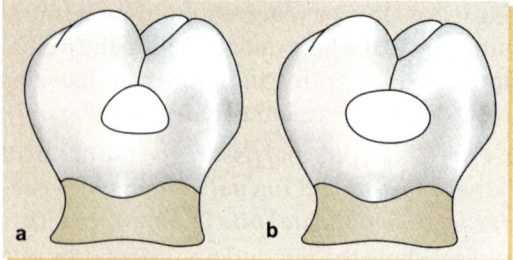

Fig. 7.8a and b: *Shapes of cavity in buccal and lingual surface*

is taken to protect the cuspal planes as far as possible, especially, the ones adjacent to the carious grooves, e.g. in case of distolingual cusp of maxillary first molars, since the cusp is small, the cutting should be carried out at the expense of the oblique ridge. In case of distal cusp of mandibular first molar, the cutting is done more at the expense of distobuccal cusp.

After preparing the occlusal cavity, keep the flat fissure bur perpendicular to the pulpal floor and move towards the buccal/lingual direction as the caries dictates. The step is prepared, keeping the bur parallel to the buccal/lingual surface.

The axial wall is placed 0.5 mm inside the dentinoenamel junction. The gingival wall is made 1.5 mm wide.

The flat gingival wall along with parallel mesial/distal walls is desirable for proper resistance form.

Similarly in case of lingual pits in the anterior teeth, the shape of the cavity can be round or oblong. The depth and walls are kept as in buccal/lingual pit cavity preparation.

Class II

The carious lesion is usually on the proximal side, which may and may not involve the occlusal surface. For gaining access, the occlusal side is to be involved.

The outline form of the occlusal part is the same as described for class I and the outline form of the proximal box is dictated by various factors viz.

 i. Extent of caries
 ii. Convexity of the proximal surfaces
 iii. Caries and plaque indices
 iv. Masticatory loads

Prepare the occlusal cavity as described earlier. Position the flat fissure bur perpendicular to the pulpal floor and extend towards the marginal ridge of the proximal area to be involved.

The isthmus width should be as narrow as possible and should not be more than 1/4th of intercuspal distance or 1.0–1.5 mm wide.

Hold the bur perpendicular to the pulpal floor and using light motion go deep slightly below the contact point and create a trough. This way, initial axial and gingival walls are created. The bur is moved buccally and lingually including the contact area. The adjacent tooth should be protected by using matrix bands.

The buccal and lingual proximal walls are kept in embrasures and meet the tangent to the respective cavosurface margin at 90° angle (Fig. 7.9).

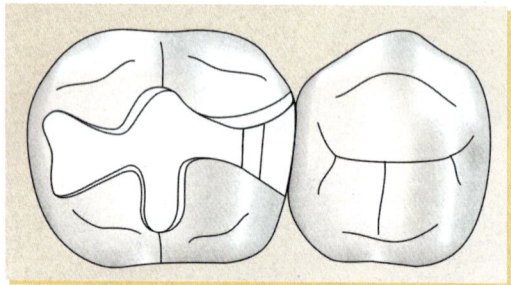

Fig. 7.9: *Buccal and lingual proximal walls kept in embrasures*

In case of maxillary teeth, mostly the molars, the contact area is more buccally, i.e. the lingual embrasures are more than the buccal embrasures. In such cases, extending the buccoproximal wall into the embrasure lead to excessive cutting of the buccal cusps. To avoid this, a reverse curve is made in the buccal proximal wall so as to have sufficient amount of dentin in that area and also to achieve butt joint with the cavosurface margins.

Such a curve, though mostly given in maxillary molars, can be given in any tooth

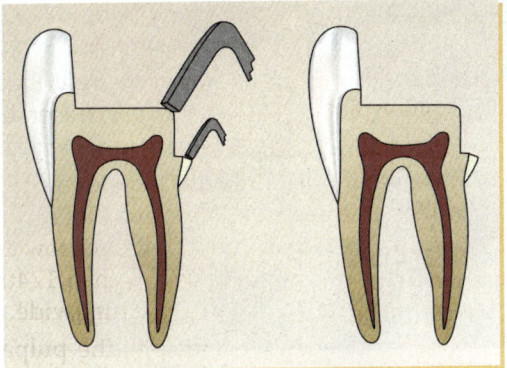

Fig. 7.10: *Beveling axiopulpal line angle and finishing gingival cavosurface margin*

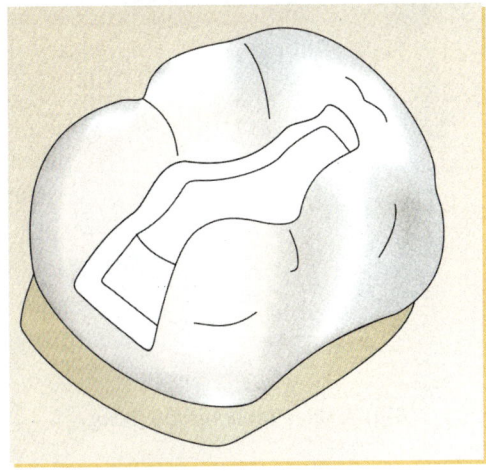

Fig. 7.11: *Proximal walls coverage occlusally to preserve marginal ridge*

where the contact area is deviated or more pronounced on one side.

The marginal trimmers are used to round off the axiopulpal line angle (Fig. 7.10).

The gingival wall should involve both enamel and dentin. The approximate width of the gingival wall is 1.0 mm or 1.5 mm if placed on enamel.

In case where the extension of gingival wall is in the cementum, the width of the gingival wall should always be less than 1.0 mm (approximately 0.7–0.8 mm).

The proximal box so formed is wider at the gingival areas as compared to the occlusal, i.e. the buccal and lingual walls are converging at the occlusal surfaces. This type of occlusal convergences contributes to the retention form. The marginal ridge is also conserved by converging the proximal walls occlusally (Fig. 7.11).

Primary resistance and retention form is achieved by the following features:

• The gingival and pulpal floor is flat and perpendicular to the long axis of the tooth.
• All walls create 90° cavosurface angle.
• Extend walls in such a way that the cusps and ridges have sufficient dentin support.
• The internal line angles are rounded off especially the axiopulpal line angle so as to have maximum bulk of silver amalgam at this area.
• Occlusal convergence of the walls.

Secondary Retentive Devices

In case, the cavity shape lacks the required retention form, extra retentive devices are utilized. This type of retention form is independent in the occlusal and the proximal areas of the cavity preparation.

The devices used for silver amalgam restorations are:
1. Slots or horizontal grooves
2. Locks or partial vertical grooves

1. Slots or Horizontal Grooves

This is a minor but definite depression in the pulpal and/or gingival wall. These are made 0.5 to 1.0 mm deep and 0.2–0.5 mm wide in dentin. In gingival wall, the slots are given 0.2 to 0.5 mm inside the dentinoenamel junction depending upon the amount of dentin available.

2. Locks or Partial Vertical Grooves

The locks are generally prepared in proximal box only.

The selection of diameter of the bur depends upon the required depth of the lock. The greater the width of the proximal box, greater would be the width of the lock (Figs 7.12 and 7.13).

Finally, the enamel margins are finished, making them straight and smooth. The

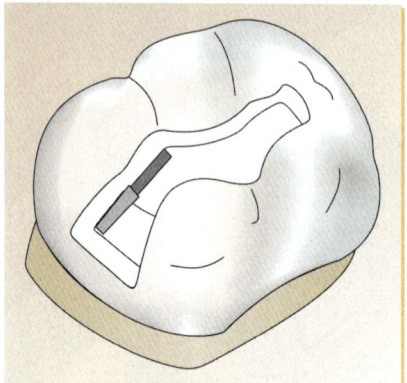

Fig. 7.12: *Preparing the locks*

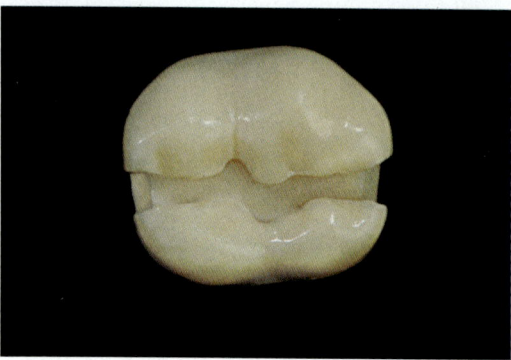

Fig. 7.14: *Mesio-occlusodistal cavity on mandibular first molar*

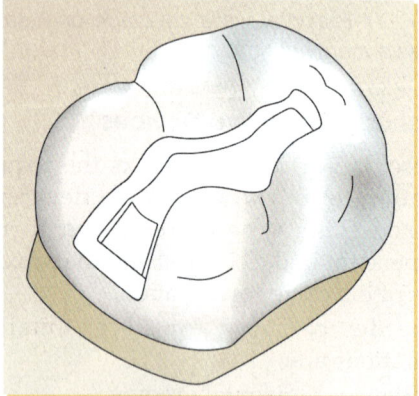

Fig. 7.13: *Prepared locks*

cavosurface angle for silver amalgam should be 90° ± 5°. The gingival wall is beveled 20° towards the cavosurface margin to ensure full-length enamel rods. This is achieved by using gingival marginal trimmers.

Modification of class II cavity (caries involving both proximal sides)

The caries involving both the proximal surfaces are commonly known as MOD preparation (Fig. 7.14). Usually two class II preparations are joined. The distal-occlusal area and the distal-proximal box is kept wider than the mesial occlusal area and the mesial proximal box. The union between these two proximal boxes at the occlusal level depends upon the remaining thickness of the connecting area and also whether this area is carious or not. In routine more than 1.0 mm area can be left without joining.

Class III

The distal surfaces of canines are the only lesions among anterior teeth which are filled with silver amalgam. Resins are usually avoided in the canines because the teeth are subjected to all three types of forces, i.e. compressive, tensile and shear.

The outline of cavity is planned in such a way so that minimal cavity cutting may be required. A small round bur, no. ½ or 1 is used to enter the carious lesion from the marginal ridge lingually. The direction of the bur is maintained perpendicular to the lingual surface of the tooth. The bur is moved 0.5 mm inside the dentinoenamel junction. The labial wall should have intact enamel as far as possible. With an inverted cone bur, the incisal and gingival walls are smoothened (Fig. 7.15). The lingual outline in such cavity preparation blends with the incisal and gingival margins,

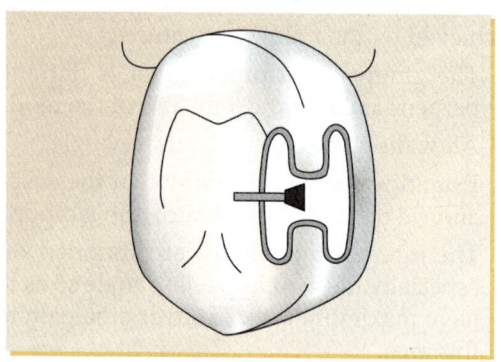

Fig. 7.15: *Smoothening incisal and gingival walls*

creating a cavity preparation without lingual proximal wall.

All cavosurface angles are 90° to the margins. The labial, incisal and gingival walls should meet the axial wall at right angle. The lingual wall, if present, may be making an obtuse angle with the axial wall (Figs 7.16 and 7.17).

Resistance form is provided by:
i. Cavosurface angle of 90°
ii. Definite internal line angles

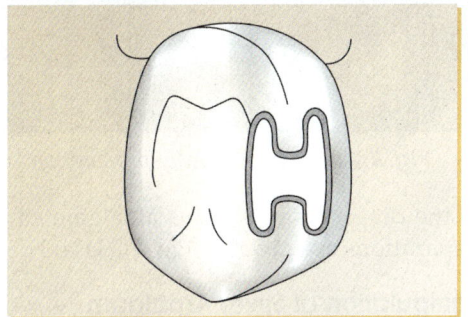

Fig. 7.16: *Class III preparation (diagrammatic)*

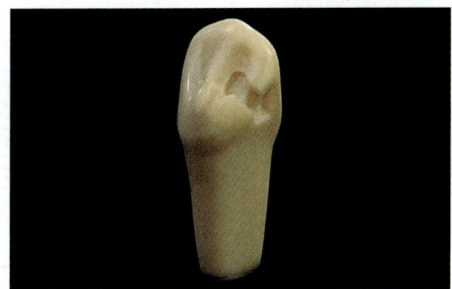

Fig. 7.17: *Lingual dovetail preparation for class III cavity preparation*

iii. Sufficient bulk of the material, i.e. adequate depth

Retention form is provided by preparing a gingival and incisal groove or undercut (Fig. 7.18). The gingival groove is place at the axiogingival line angle using small round or inverted cone bur.

Similarly the incisal groove is prepared in the incisoaxial line angle or incisoaxiolabial point angle as the shape of cavity dictates. A small round bur or inverted cone bur is utilized for purpose as described for gingival groove.

Class V

These lesions can be entirely in cementum or partially in enamel and cementum. Abrasion and erosion lesions are also very common in these areas.

The selection of the material in these areas depends upon the esthetic reasons as well as the caries index of the patient. The labial and lingual surfaces of posterior teeth can be restored with silver amalgam.

CAVITY PREPARATION

A flat fissure bur of appropriate size is used to enter the centre of the lesion at the depth of 0.5 mm inside the dentinoenamel junction. By keeping the bur perpendicular to the long axis of the tooth, the bur is directed mesially and distally and then occlusally and gingivally (Fig. 7.19). The mesial and distal extension of the preparation should be up to the line angles

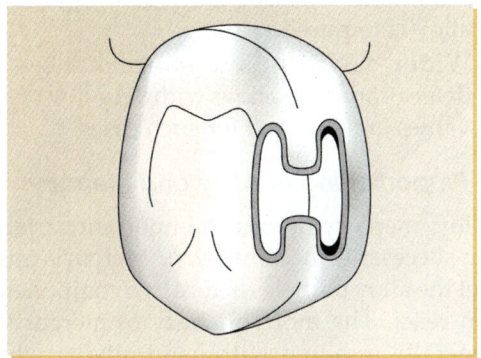

Fig. 7.18: *Gingival and incisal grooves*

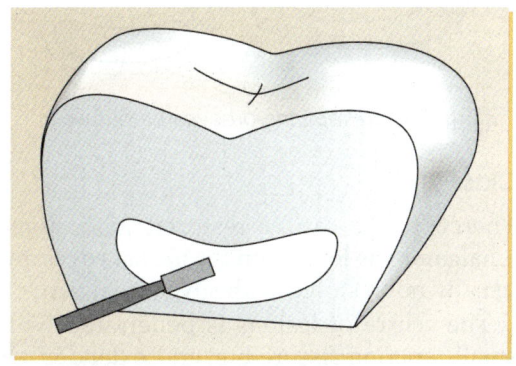

Fig. 7.19: *Preparing class V cavity*

of the tooth. The gingival wall is contoured according to the cementoenamel junction and the occlusal wall is, by and large, straight. The axial wall is also contoured mesiodistally following the outer contour of the tooth. The depth of the gingival wall is usually 0.75 mm and the occlusal wall is 1.25 mm.

All the four walls of cavity preparation, i.e. mesial, distal, occlusal and gingival diverge outward. The gingival wall, if placed in cementum is kept straight.

A small round bur (no. ¼ or ½) or inverted cone bur is used to prepare the retention grooves, one in axio-occlusal line angle directing occlusally and the other in axio-gingival line angle directing gingivally (Fig. 7.20).

In rare cases, if the cavity is extensive, the groove can be given all around the four walls of the cavity (Fig. 7.21).

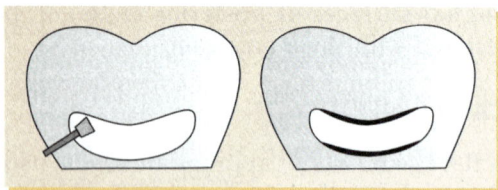

Fig. 7.20: *Preparing grooves in two line angles*

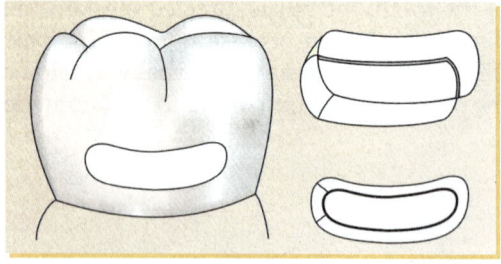

Fig. 7.21: *Preparing grooves in four walls*

Class VI

The cusp tips can be restored with silver amalgam. The lesions on the incisal edges are usually not restored with silver amalgam.

The centre of lesions is penetrated with small tapering fissure bur and extended all around to involve the caries. The depth is usually inside the dentin and the walls should have definite dentin support. A 90° cavosurface angle is prepared (Fig. 7.22). A small retentive groove using ¼ round bur or inverted cone bur can be given all around the internal line angle. The shape of the cavity is usually round.

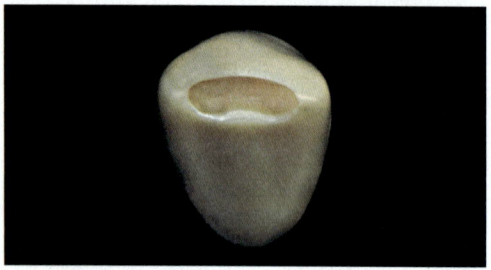

Fig. 7.22: *Class VI cavity preparation*

Line diagrams of various amalgam cavity preparations are given in Fig. 7.23a to k.

Manipulation of Silver Amalgam

The manipulation of silver amalgam involves sequence of events as follows:

1. Selection of Material

The selection of an alloy for amalgam restoration depends upon various factors keeping in mind the anatomy and pathology of the lesion. Following features are considered:

a. For restoring the areas subjected to heavy occlusal forces, an amalgam with high resistance to marginal fracture is desirable.

b. Zinc free silver alloy is preferred for areas which cannot be properly isolated.

c. For mentally retarded patients and patients with heart diseases quick setting type of alloy is required.

d. Wider cavities have more chances of deterioration, so alloys with very low creep values are required for such cases.

2. Proportioning of Alloy and Mercury

Alloy/mercury ratio is an important variable for successful manipulation. Mercury must wet the alloy particles before two components can react. The more quantity of mercury is generally required with hand mixing while low quantity of mercury is required for

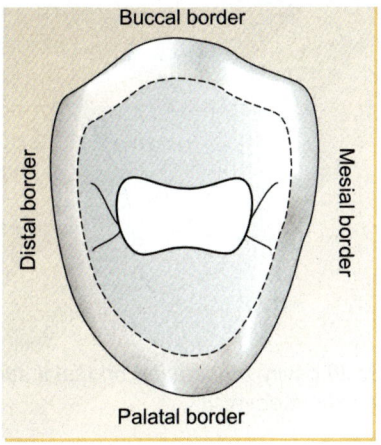

(a) Class I cavity preparation on maxillary first premolar

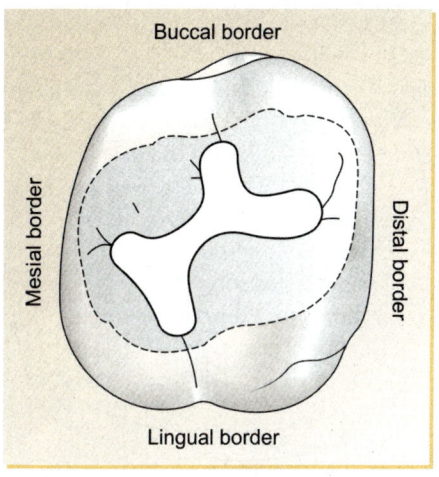

(d) Class I cavity preparation on maxillary first molar (with involving oblique ridge)

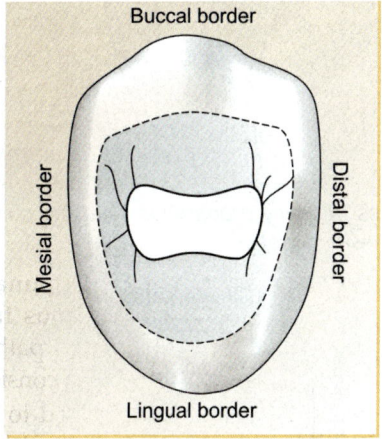

(b) Class I cavity preparation on maxillary second premolar

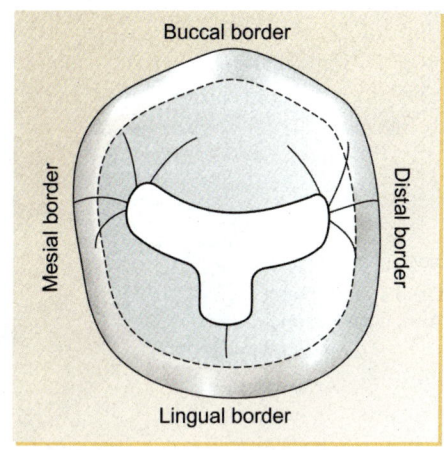

(e) Class I cavity preparation on mandibular second premolar

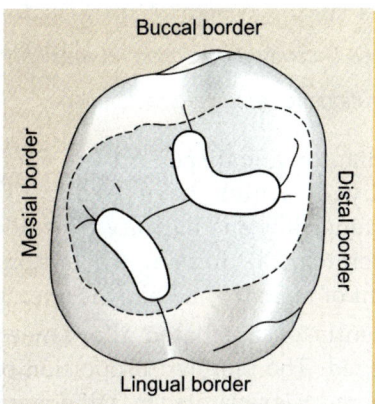

(c) Class I cavity preparation on maxillary first molar (without involving oblique ridge)

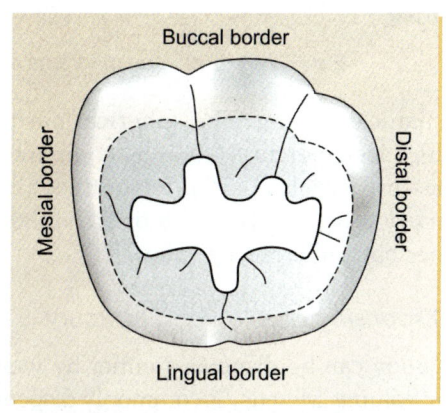

(f) Class I cavity preparation on mandibular first molar

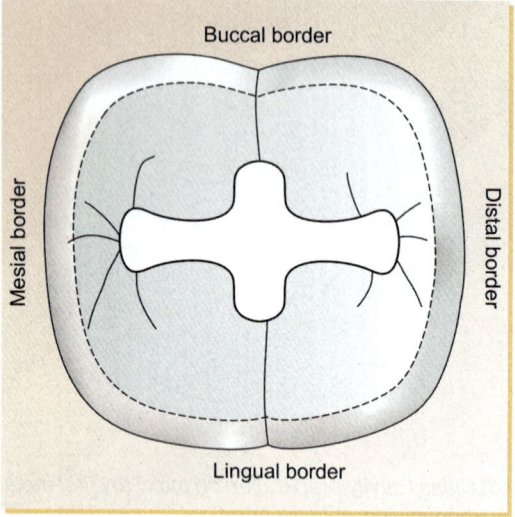

(g) Class I cavity preparation on mandibular second molar

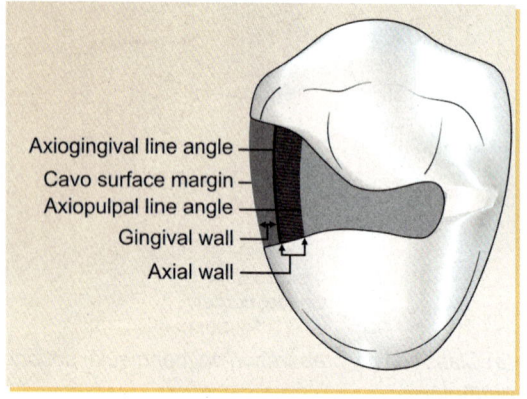

(h) Class II cavity preparation on maxillary first premolar

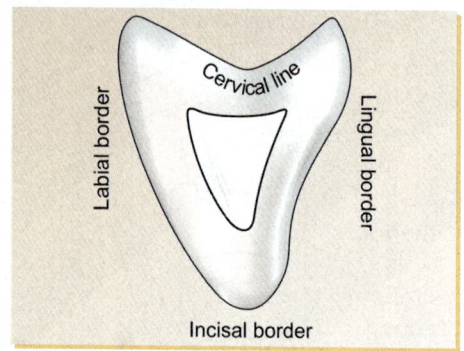

(i) Class III cavity preparation on distal surface of canine without dovetail

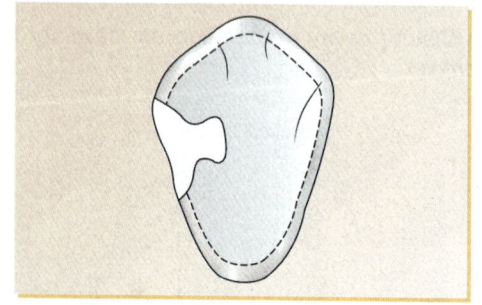

(j) Class III cavity preparation on distal surface of canine with dovetail

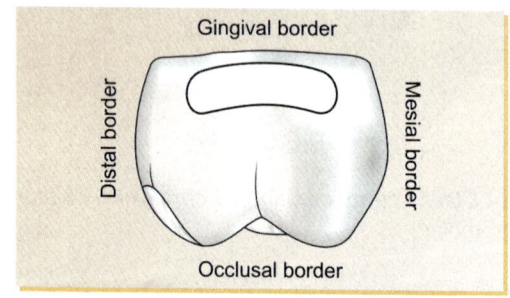

(k) Class V cavity preparation on maxillary molar

Fig. 7.23a to k: Line diagrams of cavity preparations for amalgam restoration

mechanical mixing. The spherical particles require less mercury (40%) as compared to lathe cut particles (45%). In routine, alloy/mercury ratio is kept as 5:8 or 5:7, although Eames has preferred 1:1 ratio.

3. Dispensing of Alloy and Mercury

The alloy can be dispensed either by weight or by volume. Mercury is commonly dispensed by volume.

Semiautomatic dispensers are commonly employed, which have two containers containing alloy and mercury. The ratio is set by operator. On pressing the button given amount of mercury and alloy is released.

Recently encapsulated alloy/mercury is employed. The required proportion of alloy and mercury is separated by a thin membrane. In a mechanical mixer, the membrane is broken as the mixer starts vibrating.

4. Trituration

The process of mixing of alloy with mercury is called trituration. Trituration can be carried out by hand or by mechanical amalgamators. Hand trituration is performed in glass mortar and pestle. Mechanical mixing is carried out in semi-automatic or fully automatic amalgamator.

The following factors control the quality of trituration:

   a. Time
   b. Speed
   c. Force

a. The time of trituration (6 to 20 seconds) varies depending upon the following features.

- It is higher for spherical low copper alloys and less for spherical high copper alloys.
- Types of amalgamators.
- Pestles of different weight and size.
- Increasing the size of the mix increases the mixing time.

b. The speed mostly depends upon the unit. In case of mechanical amalgamators, the speed is set by the manufacturer. In hand mixing the speed varies from operator to operator.

c. The force applied during mechanical amalgamation depends upon:

- Weight of pestle (more weight, more is force).
- Size of capsule (bigger size of capsule, so longer pestle required).
- The design of the pestle.

In hand tritutration, the operator should take the following precautions:

- The mortar should be rested on a firm base.
- Uniform pressure should be applied.
- The surface texture of pestle and mortar should be rough.
- Time should be well controlled.

Avoid excessive force; it may lead to splintering of alloy partially.

When more mass of amalgam is required for a given restoration, then a double mix should be used.

The **advantages** of mechanical amalgamator are:

- Mix is uniform.
- Trituration time is less.
- No need to squeeze excess of mercury, since the alloy/mercury ratio is proportioned by the manufacturer.

5. Mulling

After hand trituration mulling is carried out by taking mix in hand and rubbing between fingers. After mechanical trituration, mulling is carried out by rotating the mix in a pestle free capsule. It gives mix a cohesive form.

After mulling, the mass is taken in a muslin cloth and squeezed properly to remove excess mercury especially in hand trituration.

The residual mercury content affects the various properties as:

   a. Increase of residual mercury content is proportional to decrease in compressive strength.
   b. If residual mercury content increases, expansion increases.
   c. Increased creep rate.

6. Condensation

Condensation is a process by which the mix is compacted into the prepared cavity.

The aims of condensation are:

   a. Developing a continuous matrix.
   b. Removal of excess of mercury, minimizing porosity.
   c. Adapting material to all parts of the cavity walls.
   d. Better adaptation of the incremental layers of amalgam.

The condensation should be carried out as early as possible after trituration, preferably within 3–4 minutes, otherwise the mix is discarded.

Types of condensation: There are three types of condensation:

a. Hand condensation
b. Mechanical condensation
c. Ultrasonic condensation

a. Hand condensation

Hand condensers of different shapes and sizes are available to suit the cavity configuration.

The condensation should preferably start from center to periphery. The increments should be kept small. Large bulk of increments leads to air entrapment and porous and weak restoration (Fig. 7.24a and b). The cavity is overfilled slightly, which helps in burnishing and carving (Fig. 7.24c).

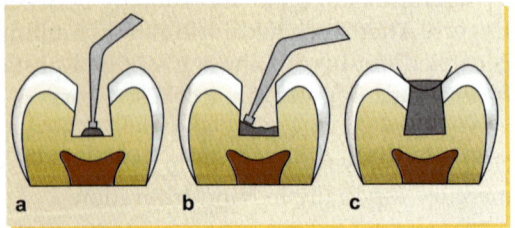

Fig. 7.24a to c: *Hand condensation. (a and b) Condensation in increments; (c) slight overfilling for burnishing*

Condensation pressure in the range of 4 to 8 lb is regarded as most appropriate. Increasing the area of condensation decreases the amount of pressure acting at the bottom of the condenser. If the forces of condensation are unduly increased, then the mass of amalgam under condenser goes along with the packing instrument rather than being adequately condensed.

After proper condensation the surface of restoration becomes shiny. This is due to accumulation of residual mercury at the surface of restoration. The residual mercury can be removed during burnishing.

Should condensers be smooth or serrated, remained controversial. Authors favoring serrated condensers are of the view that serrations make the surface of increment rough so that when next increment is added, mechanical bonding would take place. Authors favouring smooth condensers are of the view that mechanical retention is of least importance in packing various increments of amalgam mix because bonding occurs due to residual mercury which occurs at the surface of each increment.

b. Mechanical condensation

Mechanical condensation is usually avoided in routine since these instruments apply high loads, which may damage the tooth and even lead to cuspal fracture.

c. Ultrasonic condensation

Ultrasonic condensers are usually not recommended because these produce local heating of amalgam leading to release of mercury.

7. Carving, Burnishing and Initial Finishing

Carving and initial finishing is carried out to produce/simulate functional anatomy of the restoration (Fig. 7.25).

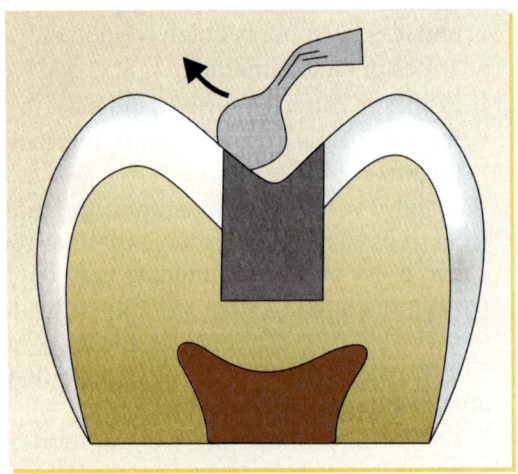

Fig. 7.25: *Initial carving and burnishing*

Carving removes excess mercury and re-establishes the contact with the opposing dentition. The alloy mass should be properly hardened before starting carving. If the mass is not set properly or is still plastic, then initiation of carving leads to pulling out of amalgam from the margins.

When scraping silver amalgam with carver, a *'ringing sound'* appears or heard that is taken as a guide for appropriate time of carving.

Carving should be carried out by keeping half of the blade of carver on tooth structure and half on restoration following the incline plane of each cusp.

Burnishing is a process in which a smooth, rigid instrument is used for smoothening restoration surface which has become rough by carving. These are conflicting views as to what should be carried out first, carving or burnishing.

Pre-carve burnishing is carried out before carving. The procedure smoothens margins and shapes the contours and curvatures.

Post-carve burnishing: After carving, the rough surface so produced is smoothened by final burnishing. At this stage, the mass is hard/set enough to prevent any disturbance of anatomy formed by carving.

8. Finishing and Polishing

Finishing involves removal of surface irregularities and to shape the restoration according to functional occlusion; whereas, polishing is the production of shiny surface which reflects light similar to enamel.

The finishing and polishing procedure tends to reduce plaque accumulation and subsequently decreases the incidence of gingival inflammation and secondary caries. The procedures provide a better marginal adaptation by removing excess amalgam from the margins that could otherwise fracture leaving a ditch between the tooth and the filling. A smooth surface produced by finishing and polishing minimizes the risk of tarnish and corrosion and is also esthetically acceptable.

After carving and burnishing, the restoration is then left undisturbed for a minimum period of 24 hours. This much time period is recommended to allow for setting, hardening and dimensional changes in amalgam. The patient is cautioned not to chew from that area for a period of 7–8 hours.

As the material sets, the surface of the restoration becomes rough due to the heterogenous structure of amalgam on setting. Finishing is now begun with the use of steel finishing burs or stones. Finishing of cervical areas is carried out by inserting fine water resistant strips cervical to the contact area through the interdental space and moving them to and fro.

The abrasives during finishing should be applied in a descending grade, i.e. coarse, medium, fine and ultra fine. The final polish or the metallic luster is obtained by application of a suitable polishing agent like tin oxide, zinc oxide, chalk, pumice, extra fine silex, etc. carried with a soft rotating brush or rubber cup. For polishing in the contact areas and gingival embrasures, the abrasive is introduced through polishing strips.

During polishing, the restoration should be kept moist and only low rotational speeds with light intermittent pressure should be used to avoid any overheating. Excessive heat can damage the pulp and also tends to bring mercury to the surface.

With the advent of high copper amalgams, it is now possible to finish the restorations much earlier. It is an established fact that the high copper alloys can be polished 15–30 minutes after condensation. High copper amalgams have a rapid setting tendency and achieve high early compressive strength, allowing them to withstand the forces of finishing quite earlier.

A few authors are of the view that polishing of high copper amalgam is less important than conventional amalgam, because the former is less susceptible to tarnish and marginal breakdown.

Hazards during finishing and polishing of amalgam restorations:
• Production of aerosols
• High temperatures may damage pulp, bring mercury to the surface and produce mercury vapours.

8

Cavity Preparation for Cast Inlays

The operator, in routine, is confronted in many occasions where restoration with silver amalgam is not feasible and advisable. In these cases cast restorations are indicated, which can be inlays, onlays and full crowns fabricated from precious or base metal alloys. The inlay, by definition, is the intracoronal restoration which involves occlusal and/or proximal surfaces without involving the cusps. The onlay is the restoration which along with inlay covers one or more cusps but not all. The full crown covers all the cusps. Although various alloys are being used for casting; however, for the beginners, cavity preparation for gold alloys is described here.

Indications

- When superior control over contacts and contours is required.
- To some extent for modification of contacts and contours.
- To modify the embrasure area so as to minimize periodontal problems.
- Where better strength of the restoration is required.
- Where proper dimensions of inclined planes are desirous for better functional occlusion.

Contraindication

- In deciduous and developing teeth.
- Where the patient exhibits high caries risk.
- Where the patient has silver restoration in their teeth

- Occlusal disharmony, if any, should be corrected prior to gold inlay restoration

Advantages

- Coefficient of thermal expansion is better in cast alloy than silver amalgam, so physically preferred.
- Wear resistance is high; gold castings maintain marginal integrity for many years.
- Provides proper anatomical form.
- Do not discolor the tooth (no tarnish and corrosion).
- It can be finished and polished in much better way than other restorative materials.
- It is biocompatible.
- The gold alloy does not fracture in function.
- Esthetically better.

Disadvantages

- Not a tooth colored material
- Cement lining between tooth and restoration leads to marginal leakage
- Expensive
- Patient visits are increased

CAVITY PREPARATION

Prior to cavity preparation, the tooth must be evaluated carefully for the following factors that influence the design of the cavity.
- The length of the clinical crown.
- The anatomic characteristics of the occlusal, proximal, buccal and lingual surfaces.

- The position of the tooth in the arch.
- The occlusal and proximal relationships.
- Unusual esthetic problems.
- The relationship and condition of the soft tissues.
- The extent and the location of the carious lesions.

Armamentarium

- No. 271 carbide bur
- No.169L carbide bur
- Spoon excavator
- Enamel hatchet
- Gingival marginal trimmer

Principles of Cavity Preparation

The basic principles of Dr GV Black are followed for cast inlay preparation.

I. Outline Form

i. External outline form

The external outline form of the cavity preparation for gold inlay should have straight lines and smooth flowing curves, avoiding any sharp angles. The finishing line should be extended on the occlusal surface to include retentive fissures. On the proximal and cervical areas, the carious lesion is removed and the margins are placed which provide convenience for finishing. Enamel that has been undermined by caries is removed. In order to obtain a well-fitted casting, the cavosurface margin is placed on sound, tooth surface.

The placement of bevels makes the outline form slightly wider for cast restorations (Fig. 8.1a to c).

ii. Internal outline form

The pulpal floor and the axial wall of the gold inlay preparation must be placed in the dentin. When the preparation has to be taken beyond its usual internal limits because of the extent of the lesion or injury, the additional loss of dentin is replaced with an appropriate cement base. The 2°–5° taper required normally varies with the depth of the preparation. The taper should not be visible to the eye. In shallow

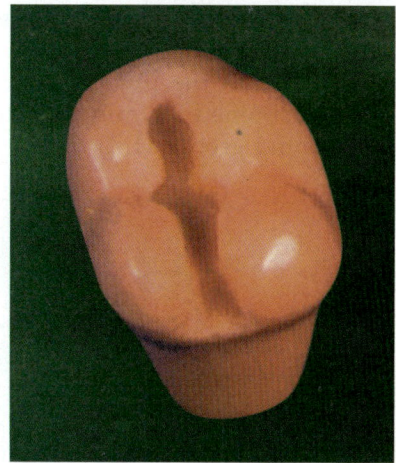

Fig. 8.1a: *Class II cavity preparation for cast gold—occlusal view*

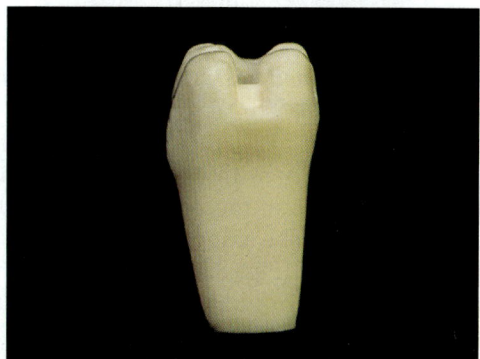

Fig. 8.1b: *Proximal view*

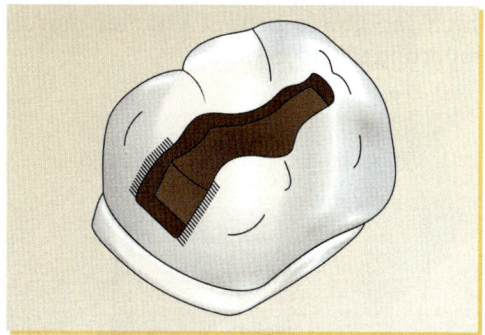

Fig. 8.1c: *Diagrammatic representation (dotted lines indicate secondary flare)*

preparations, parallelism enhances the resistance and retention form. Deep cavities require taper to facilitate seating of the restoration.

Since the exact measurement for the length of the occlusal walls is difficult, it is recommended that the pulpal floor will usually be positioned 0.5 mm into dentin below the central groove (1.75 to 2.00 mm) (Fig. 8.2).

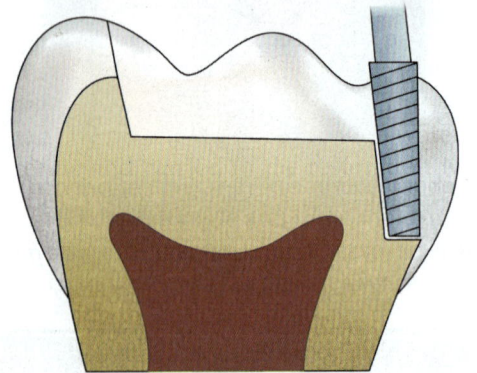

Fig. 8.2: *Occlusal and axial walls are in dentin with slight taper of the axial wall*

Line angles in both the occlusal and proximal portions of the preparation should be well defined. The axiopulpal line angle is slightly rounded (Fig. 8.3). The flare of the proximal walls should form axioproximal angles of 100 to 110 degrees.

All questionable grooves and fissures should be included. The bur is inclined at the marginal ridge area so as to create long taper, which facilitates proper enamel margins supporting sound dentin.

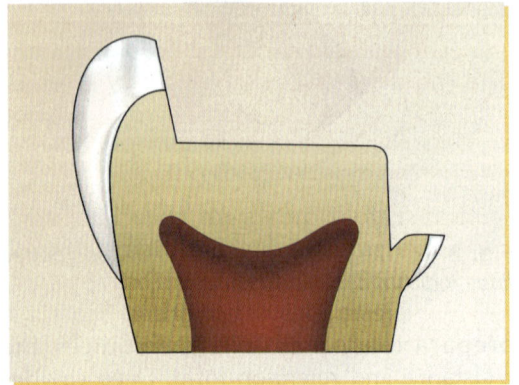

Fig. 8.3: *Rounded axiopulpal line angle and reverse bevel at the gingival wall*

II. Resistance and Retention Forms

Lateral or tangential forces usually cause displacement of the restoration unless adequate resistance and retention have been incorporated in the preparation. Frictional retention can be achieved by the action of dentin and enamel walls grasping the restoration (intracoronal retention). Most dental cements are not adhesive. The strength of the cement bond alone will not provide retention for the casting. Cement provides only a moderate mechanical lock between the minute irregularities of the cavity walls and the casting surface.

Inlay Taper

A basic requirement of the cavity preparations for the cast gold inlay is that the cavity walls should diverge occlusally from the floor of the preparation.

The preparation has a line of draw that describes the path of insertion and removal of the casting, which determines the axis of taper. The axis of taper for a class I and class II preparation generally parallels the long axis of the tooth; for a class V, axis of taper generally is perpendicular to the long axis of the tooth.

Ideally no taper is advisable; however, a range between 4 and 6° is used because it provides adequate retention of the cemented casting. The axial length of the preparation will influence the amount of taper. Longer preparations need more taper than shorter preparations. The degree of taper should not be so great so as to lose the frictional grasp between tooth and the restoration. It must however be sufficient to allow the complete seating of the restoration in the cavity.

Pulpal and cervical floors ideally should be perpendicular to the lines of force that will influence the restoration. Floors positioned perpendicular to these lines of force absorbs the stress over a broad area of tooth.

Well-defined line angles are also important in obtaining resistance and retention form. The axiopulpal line angle is slightly rounded to dissipate the stresses.

The occlusal interlock or dovetail is a major factor in resistance and retention form.

Tapered grooves extending from cervical floor to the occlusal surface, are sometimes placed in the dentin portion of the proximal walls which aid in preventing lateral dislodgement of the restoration (Fig. 8.4).

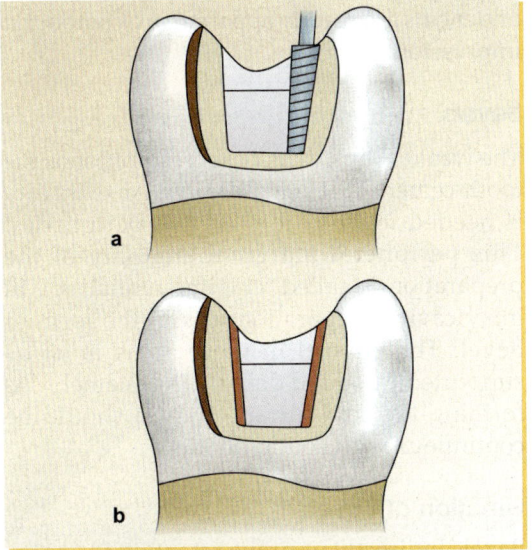

Fig. 8.4: *Proximal grooves are incorporated to improve retention form. (a) preparing grooves with tapering fissure bur, (b) prepared grooves*

Factors Affecting Retention of Cast Restorations

Many factors control the dislodging forces vis-à-vis aid in retention of the restoration. The following factors affect the retention of cast inlays:

1. *Magnitude of the dislodging forces:* The quantum of vertical and oblique forces tends to dislodge the restoration. The magnitude of the dislodging forces depends on the stickiness of food and forces generated due to occluding and lateral movement of the jaws. The tilting forces are more affective than the vertical ones.
2. *Geometry of the tooth preparation:* The geometric form of the preparation is very important since the cements may not provide necessary retention. This is because most of the traditional cements are non-adhesive, i.e. they act by increasing the frictional resistance between tooth and restorations.

   The geometrical forms generally responsible for retention are:
   a. *Taper:* Ideally parallel walls provide best retention; however, a slight taper is necessary for the fabrication of wax pattern. As long as this taper is small, the movement of the cemented restora-tion will be effectively restrained by limited path of withdrawal. As the taper increases, there will be free movement of the restoration along the path of withdrawal.
   b. *Surface area:* Restorations with long axial walls are more retentive than those with short axial walls, e.g. restorations for molars are more retentive than for premolars.
   c. *Stress concentration:* It is established that when a retentive failure occurs, it occurs due to cohesive failure in the cement layer. These stresses are not uniform and may be concentrated around the junction of the axial and occlusal surfaces.
   d. *Type of preparation:* The grooves in a preparation with a limited path of withdrawal do not markedly affect its retention; however, where the addition of a groove limits the path of withdrawal, retention is increased.
3. *Roughness of the surfaces being cemented:* The retention of rough surfaces is more; so roughness can be artificially created using alumina particles on inner side of the inlays.
4. *Materials being cemented:* The more reactive the alloy is, the better will be the adhesion with the luting cement. Therefore, base metal alloys are better retained than less reactive gold metals.
5. *Type of luting agent:* The adhesive resin cements are more retentive than conventional cements.

III. Removing Carious Dentin

The remaining caries is removed and after removal, the floors and the walls are carefully evaluated. Decision is to be taken whether small undermined area can be filled or the preparation is to be modified for onlays.

IV. Convenience Form

Convenience form provides the required accessibility and visibility. The taper and flare of proximal walls are examples of convenience form, since they aid in bevel placement and also finishing and polishing.

V. Finishing Enamel Walls and the Margins

The conventional cutting instruments leave roughened surfaces. Even hand instruments may leave notched irregularities on walls and margins. The marginal fit of a gold restoration depends upon the approximation of cast metal to tooth tissue, which should be smooth.

Whenever a direct wax pattern is to be formed, the bevel used is of great bulk and extends a greater width across the cervical floor. The bevel on the cervical margin should be uniform about ¼ to ⅓ of mesiodistal width of the cervical floor. Such a bevel is placed with a gingival marginal trimmer prior to finishing the proximal enamel walls (Fig. 8.5).

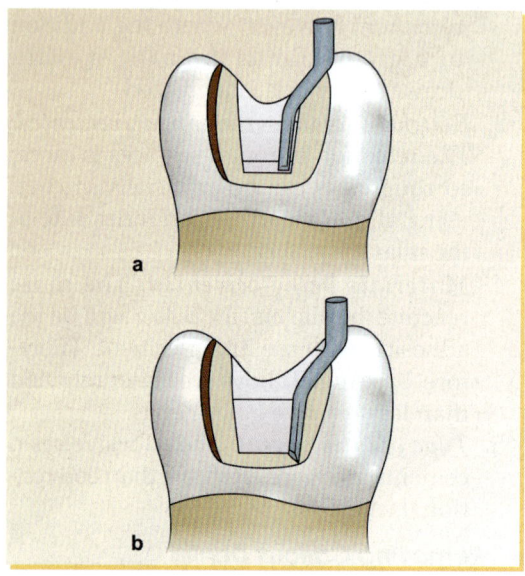

Fig. 8.5: *(a) Gingival marginal trimmer used for finishing cervical wall, (b) gingival marginal trimmer used for making cervical cavosurface bevel*

VI. Cleaning and Critical Appraisal of the Cavity

The cavity after preparation is cleaned with water and scrutinized carefully for any imperfections. A trial impression with gutta-percha or impression compound is always helpful to evaluate taper and the line of draw of the preparation. Even relatively minute under cuts are readily apparent in a compound impression.

Bevels

The weakest link in any cast restoration is the tooth-cement-cast joint complex. An extra care is needed to prepare marginal peripheries. This peripheral marginal anatomy of the preparation is called 'circumferential tie'. In inlay cavity preparation it is in the form of bevel. The enamel in these areas must be supported by sound dentin. The enamel rods forming the cavosurface margin should be continuous with sound dentin.

Function of Bevels

Bevels indirectly improve retention forms for a cast restoration since bevels decrease the direct frictional component between the tooth and the casting. The circumferential tie of tooth-casting interphase is a susceptible friction zone and if left to direct contact will lead to less retention of the restoration.

The different types of bevels are:

1. *Partial:* It involves part of enamel wall (Fig. 8.6a). This is indicated in direct filling gold.

2. *Short:* In involves entire enamel wall (Fig. 8.6b). This type of bevel best suited in cast gold inlays.

3. *Inverted:* It is given on the labial shoulder of metal ceramic crowns to effectively improve the esthetics at the margins (Fig. 8.6c).

4. *Reverse bevel:* This bevel is placed at the dentinal portion of the cervical wall towards the axiopulpal line angle. This is indicated in cast gold inlay preparations (Fig. 8.6d).

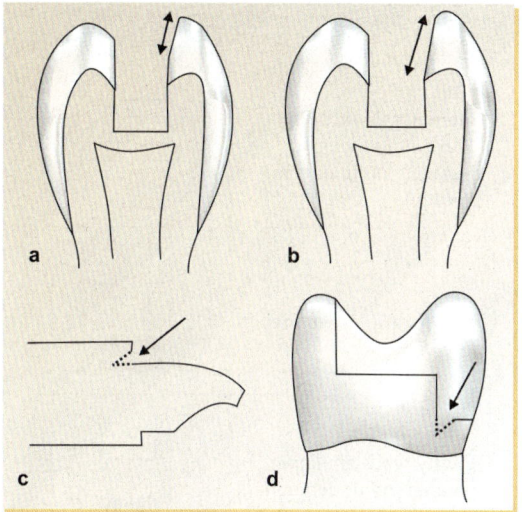

Fig. 8.6: *Types of bevel. (a) Partial bevel, (b) short bevel, (c) inverted bevel, (d) reverse bevel*

The Flares

The flares can be of following types:

a. *The primary flare:* As per the old concept of inlay cavity preparation, the proximal walls were divided into two halves. The axial half was placed at 90° to the axial wall and proximal half had an angulation of 45° to the axial half. This proximal half that helped to bring the proximal wall into self cleansing areas was known as the primary flare (Fig. 8.7a—old concept)

It was believed that the axial wall should be at 90° to the axial wall to provide the retention and resistance form to the cavity but later it was found that flaring of the walls right from axiofacial or axiolingual line angles till the cavosurface margin did not alter the retention and resistance form. This implies that the flaring of lingual wall and buccal wall of proximal box from the axial wall (axiolingual and axiofacial line angles respectively) to the proximal cavosurface margins is known as primary flare (Fig. 8.7 b—present concept)

Functions: The function of the primary flare is to keep the proximal, buccal and lingual walls in the self-cleansing areas.

b. *The secondary flare:* The secondary flare is a flat plane superimposed peripherally to a primary flare. It is as good as the occlusal bevel given to create a circumferential tie in gold inlays to take the advantage of malleability of gold alloys (Fig. 8.7b).

However, if the proximal wall extend the stipulated angulation as mentioned (may be because of broad contact area or iatrogenic), then the operator will have to analyse the involvement of the incline plane of respective cusps. If more than 1/3rd of the incline plane of the cusp is involved then, cusp coverage is recommended (Fig. 8.7 c).

Functions: A secondary flare creates the needed obtuse angulation of the marginal tooth structure given exclusively for gold inlay preparations.

Line diagrams of various cavity preparation for gold inlay are given in Fig. 8.8a to g.

The difference in cavity preparation for silver amalgam and cast restoration is given in Table 8.1.

FINISHING AND POLISHING

Initial finishing of a gold inlay is carried out mostly in the laboratory. The casting is separated from the investment and cleaned using brush or steam. It is critical to examine the casting carefully, preferably with a magnifying glass, for any defects such as nodules or voids and even for any adherent investment before it is tried onto the die. Nodules or blebs are removed carefully with chisels or small burs. The casting is then pickled in 50% hydrochloric acid and neutralized in sodium bicarbonate. Initially, the sprue serves as a handle and helps in manipulating its insertion and removal. The sprue is then separated as close to the surface as possible using a separating disk. The stub of the sprue is smoothened.

Any obvious extension of the casting beyond the margins is removed up to the finish line with a small cylindrical point rotating away from the operator. Occlusal surface is then finished using abrasive stones and discs in an order of descending abrasiveness.

Table 8.1: *Differences in cavity preparation for silver amalgam and cast restoration*

Silver amalgam	Cast restoration
1. Intercuspal width is 1/4th of intercuspal distance (outline form is narrow)	Intercuspal width is 1/3rd of intercuspal distance (outline form is wide)
2. Cavity depth is more	Comparatively less depth
3. Cavity walls are kept convergent occlusally (minor undercuts)	Cavity walls are kept parallel (no undercuts)
4. Buccal and lingual proximal walls are convergent occlusally	Buccal and lingual proximal walls are parallel
5. Cavosurface bevel is contraindicated (butt joint is preferred)	Cavosurface bevel is given
6. All line angles and point angles are rounded and axiopulpal line angle is bevelled	All line angles and point angles are well defined and axiopulpal line angle is slightly rounded
7. No reverse bevel is given	Reverse bevel is indicated
8. Grooves are not given, only locks are given	Grooves are given, locks are not given

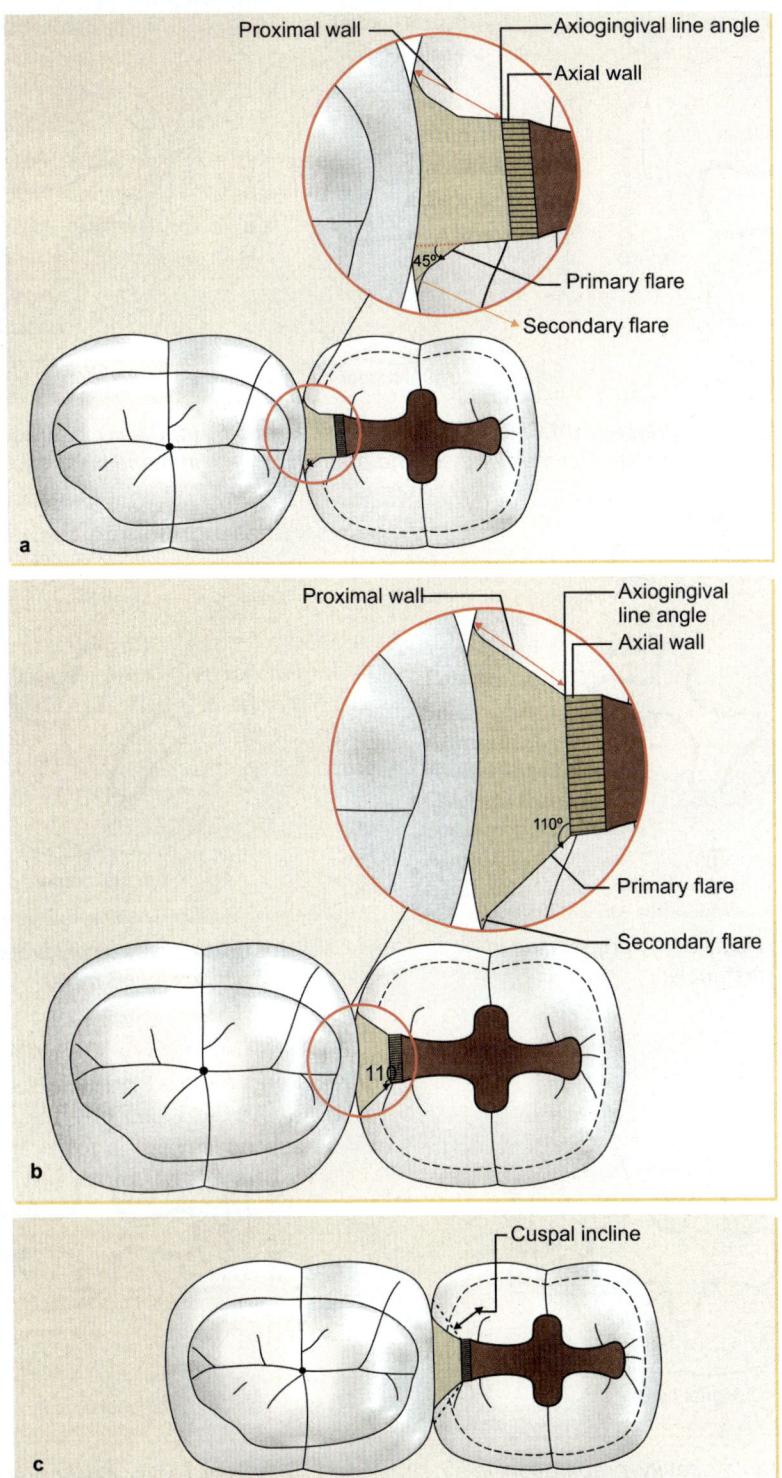

Fig. 8.7a to c: *(a) Old concept of inlay cavity preparation, (b) present concept of inlay cavity preparation, (c) extension of proximal wall in broad contact areas*

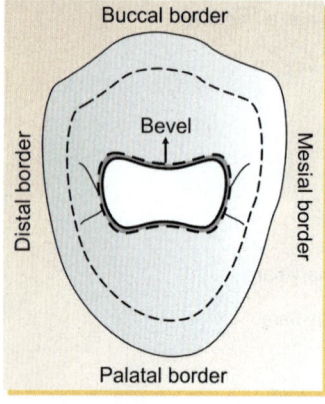

(a) Class I inlay cavity preparation in maxillary first premolar

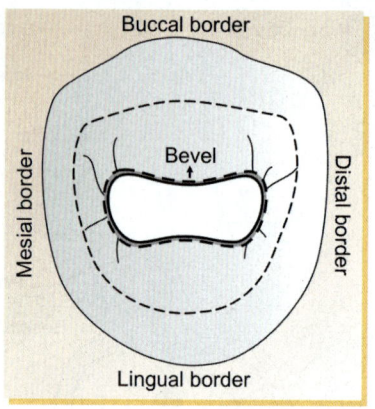

(b) Class I inlay cavity preparation in maxillary second premolar

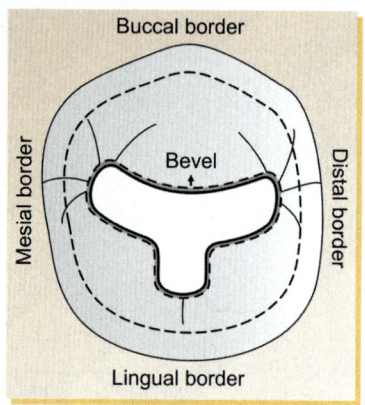

(c) Class I inlay cavity preparation in mandibular second premolar

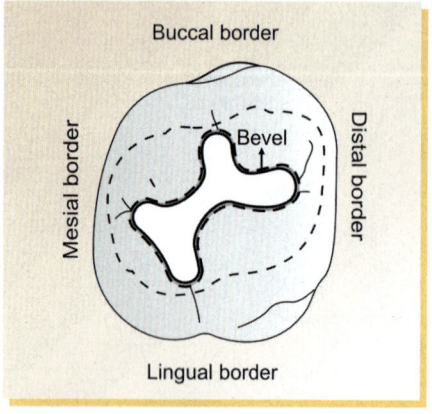

(d) Class I inlay cavity preparation in maxillary first molar

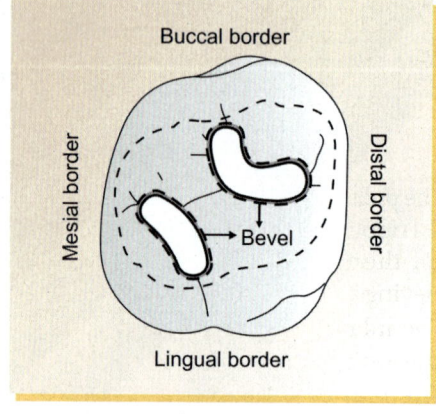

(e) Class I inlay cavity preparation in maxillary second molar

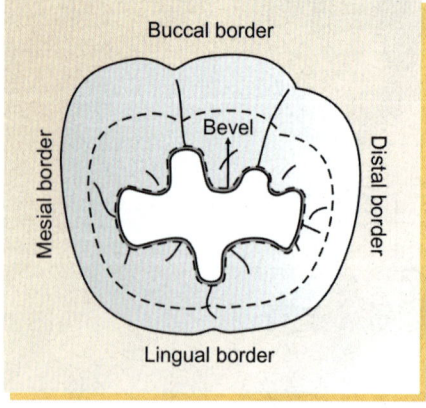

(f) Class I inlay cavity preparation in mandibular first molar

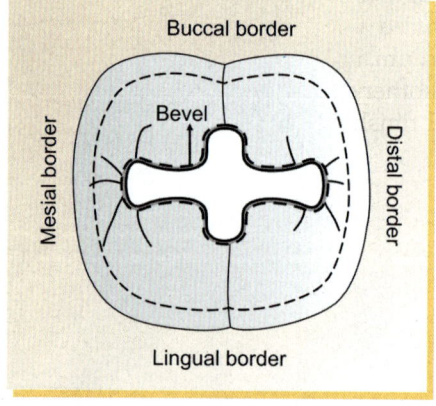

(g) Class I inlay cavity preparation in mandibular second molar

Fig. 8.8a to g: Line diagram of cavity preparation for gold inlay

The proximal surface is contoured lightly with a $\frac{1}{2}'' - \frac{5}{8}''$ carborundum disk followed by smoothening with paper disks.

The occlusion is checked with an articulating paper, and premature contacts, if any, are refined by selective grinding. The roughness so created is finished with a fine rubber polishing points (Fig. 8.9).

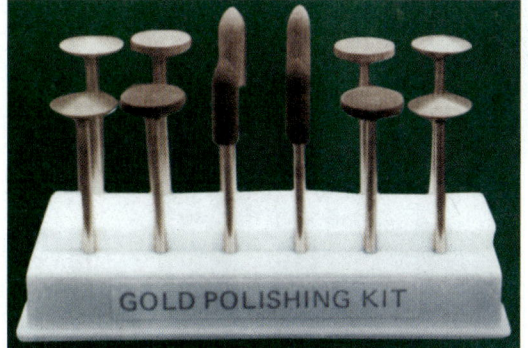

Fig. 8.9: *Gold polishing kit*

The polishing is carried out using bristle brush and Tripoli. The brush should always be moved from the casting to the tooth surface. For achieving a very high luster, rouge may be used.

The inlay is seated into the cavity and the occlusion is checked intraorally.

The marginal relationships are checked under a magnifying glass by running a probe across the metal tooth interface. In cases where the margins of the inlay are bulky or override the unprepared tooth surfaces, the excess is reduced with a carborundum disk, stone or medium and fine cuttle disks. The surfaces are smoothened with pre-shaped fine grit stones and finished with fine waterproof disks. All those areas that have been adjusted intra-orally are polished again.

The inlay is now cemented in the cavity and burnished.

COMPOSITE INLAY

Despite the incremental build up and techniques, polymerization shrinkage is a major problem that contributes to failure of composite restorations. To overcome clinical problems, the indirect composite system was introduced which has demonstrated dramatic improvement in clinical performance. A composite inlay is defined as a restoration which is cemented into a cavity prepared specifically for the composite material. A solid mass simulating the cavity shape is fabricated from composite resin outside the oral cavity.

Cavity Preparation Features

- *Taper:* 8–10 degree
- *Minimum depth:* 1.5 mm
- *Isthmus width:* 2.0 mm
- No cavosurface bevel
- No undercuts in the preparation

CERAMIC INLAY

The use of porcelains in constructing individual inlays and crowns started in late 1800s. The ceramic inlay provides best esthetics, a good marginal fit, retention, sealing, fracture resistance and shade matching. Ceramic inlays are a viable alternative to conventional restorations.

Cavity design: Same features as composite inlays except depth is more.

9

Fabrication of Cast Inlays

The fabrication of inlays is carried out in laboratory. The procedure involves many steps and each step is important for the success of the treatment.

The steps involved are:

A. IMPRESSION TECHNIQUE

An impression is a negative replica of any object. In dentistry, impression is the negative replica of teeth and the surrounding tissues. From this negative form of the teeth and the surrounding structures, a positive reproduction, known as cast, is made.

Several types of impression materials are available with varying degree of accuracy. Most of newly available materials have excellent accuracy and are used in routine.

The impression can be made on prefabricated tray or the tray can be fabricated outside the oral cavity.

i. *Selection of the impression tray:* The stock trays (Fig. 9.1) are used for reversible hydrocolloid; whereas custom trays (Fig. 9.2) are used for polysulphide and polyether impression materials.

Custom trays are usually preferred because they allow a more uniform, thin layer of 2.0–3.0 mm of the impression material. A uniform thickness of impression material will lead to less distortion. Elastomeric impression materials in thicknesses greater than 3.0 mm show greater shrinkage and

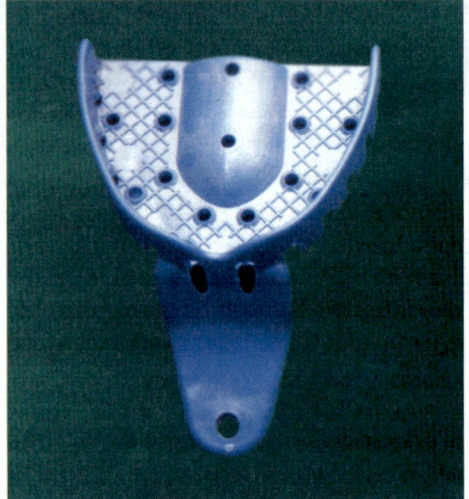

Fig. 9.1: *Stock tray*

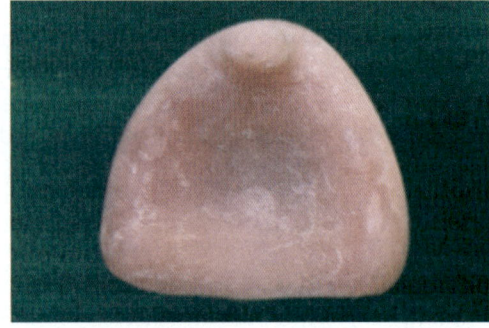

Fig. 9.2: *Custom tray*

distortion. Thickness of less than 2.0 mm would either tear or distort easily.

ii. *Fabrication of custom tray:* Acrylic resin is used to form a custom tray. A study model provides the basis for forming the tray. The study model is covered with base plate wax and trimmed so that it extends 2.0–3.0 mm beyond the necks of the teeth. A horseshoe shaped form is used for both articles. The diagnostic cast must be covered with tin foil before the wax is adapted. A 3.0 × 3.0 mm hole is cut through the wax over the posterior teeth on both sides and in the incisor area (Fig. 9.3).

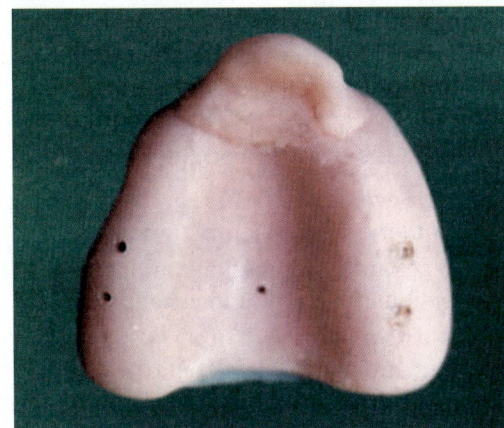

Fig. 9.4: *Fabrication of custom tray (making perforation)*

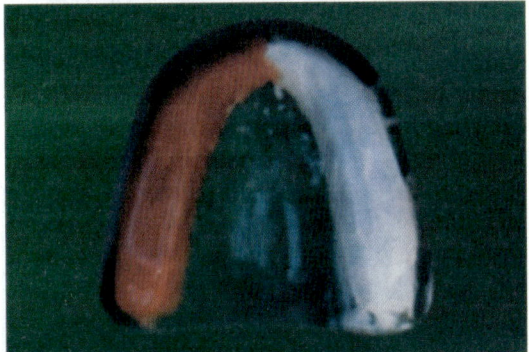

Fig. 9.3: *Fabrication of custom tray (filling undercuts)*

Before the resin tray is made, the wax is covered by a layer of tin foil to prevent the wax from impregnating the surface of the tray using the exothermic polymerization of the resin.

The cold cure acrylic resin is mixed and allowed to stand till the dough stage is reached. It is then rolled to form a horseshoe shape and flattened. A small handle is placed in the middle. Lateral extensions can be made for easy removal. When the tray is hard, but still warm to touch, it is removed from the cast and the tin foil is peeled off. The tray should be prepared at least six hours prior to making the final impression. The tray is then coated with the tray adhesive. Different tray adhesives are available. Small perforations can be created which enhance the adhesion of impression material (Fig. 9.4).

iii. *Making the impression:* The impression material is mixed following manufacturers'

instructions. Usually powder-liquid or two paste system materials are available. The impression after setting is removed in vertical directions (Fig. 9.5). Thereafter, it is washed and dried. It is poured with adequate gypsum material to form a cast and die.

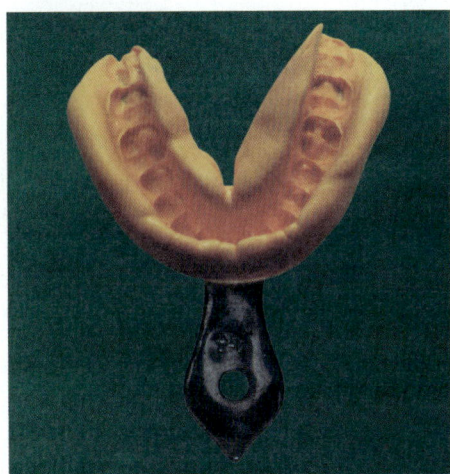

Fig. 9.5: *Final impression*

B. CONSTRUCTION OF THE DIE AND THE WORKING MODEL

A 'Die' is the positive replica of one tooth whereas cast is of the whole arch. Usually the prepared tooth is separated from the cast (die making) and the rest of the procedures are carried out on the die.

The 'dies' can be constructed in two ways.

I. Techniques utilizing two sets of pours

II. Techniques utilizing one set of pour

I. Techniques Utilizing Two Sets of Pours

- Two or even more pours can be had using elastomeric impression materials
- Two separate impressions are required if reversible hydrocolloid is used.

Dies are prepared from the first pour. Working models poured from the second impression (or obtained from second pour of the same impression depending upon the impression material) are used for articulation on which wax pattern contacts, contours and occlusal morphology is built. The dies are reserved for final margination, detail adjustments, surface treatment and spring of the wax pattern.

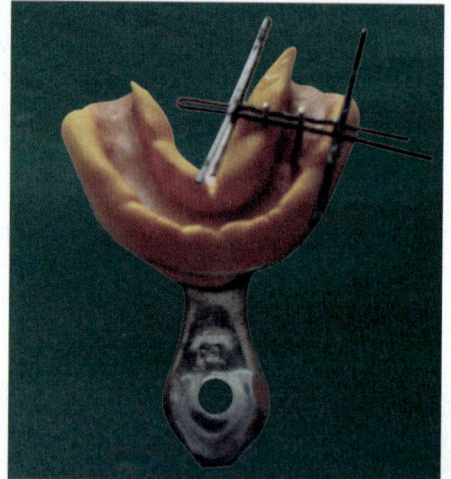

Fig. 9.6: *Stabilizing the die pin*

Advantages

- The mounted casts are not subjected to distortion.
- There is complete immobilization during building the wax pattern.

Disadvantages

- Moving the wax pattern from the working model to the die and vice-versa can induce stresses in the wax.
- The two replicas of the tooth may not have exactly the same dimensions, which induce stresses in the wax pattern.

II. Techniques Utilizing One Set of Pour (Cast)

In this technique, the die will be part of the working cast (Figs 9.6 to 9.12). The die can be removed from the working cast to draw and shape the wax pattern.

Advantages

- It saves time.
- It eliminates dimensional discrepancies between dies.
- There is less distortion of the wax pattern.

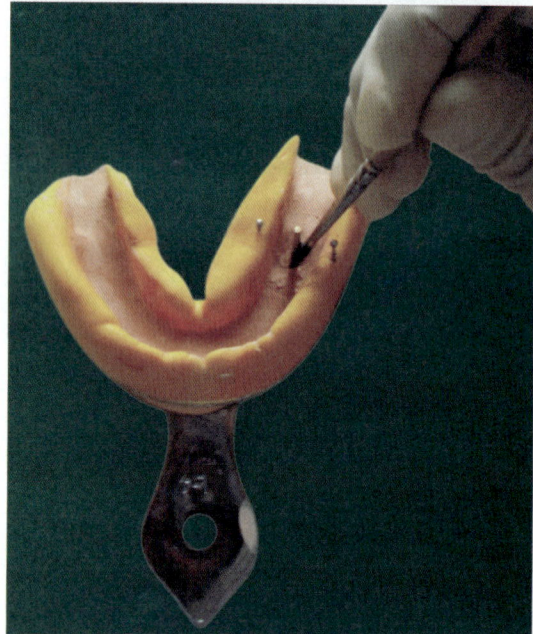

Fig. 9.7: *Adjusting the pin in initial pour*

Disadvantages

- Manipulation is difficult.
- Necessity for additional equipment.

Materials used for Die Fabrication

Various materials have been used for construction of dies. The basic requirements for such materials are:

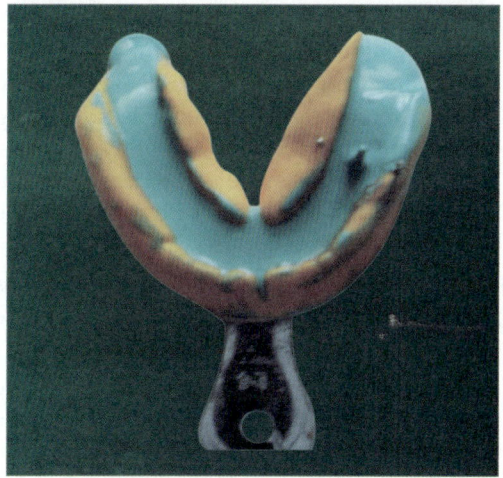

Fig. 9.8: *Die pin set in final pour*

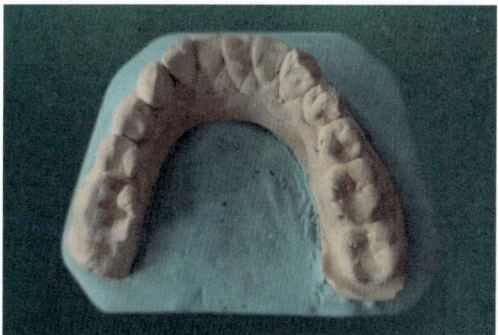

Fig 9.9: *Prepared cast*

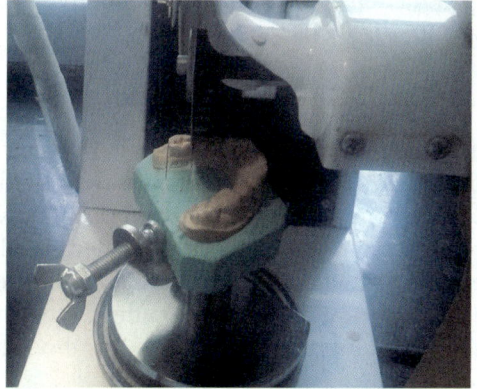

Fig. 9.10: *Cutting die with die cutter*

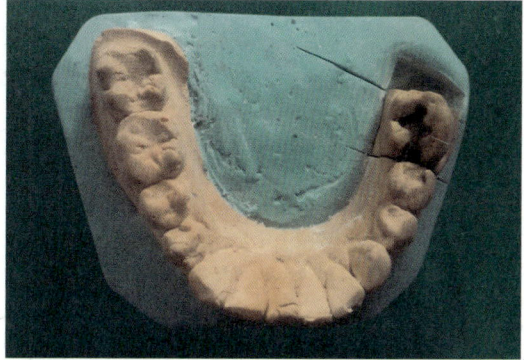

Fig 9.11: *Die after cutting*

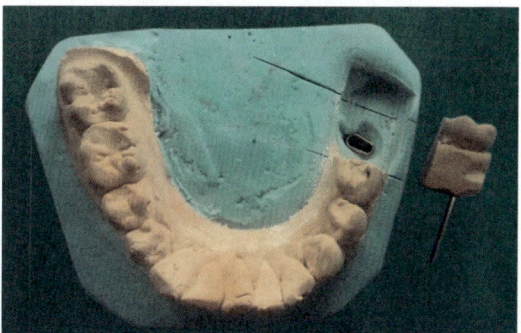

Fig 9.12: *Cast and die*

- It should be compatible with the impression material.
- It should be dimensionally stable.
- It should have a smooth, non-abradable surface.
- It should be able to accommodate auxiliary pins, if required.
- It should also be able to receive a spacer to create space for the luting agent.

The materials used for construction of dies are:

1. **Gypsum (dental stone):** Type IV and type V dental stone are the commonly used materials. The physical properties are tabulated in Table 9.1.

Manipulation can vary the strength. Decreasing the water/powder ratio increases the strength. Increasing the mixing time will

Table 9.1: Physical properties of gypsum				
Properties	Water/Powder ratio	Setting time (min.)	Setting expansion (%)	Compressive strength (psi)
Type IV	0.22–0.24	12±4	0.00 – 0.10	5000
Type V	0.18–0.22	12±4	0.10 – 0.30	7000

increase the strength (in limits). The incorpora-tion of amalgam powder may increase strength. Incorporation of accelerators and retarders cause a loss of strength.

Setting time can be accelerated by the operator by use of fine particle gypsum, low water/powder ratio, long and fast mixing, use of 3.0% potassium sulphate solution or the use of slurry water. The use of slurry water is the safest method.

2. **Electroformed dies:** Certain metals can be electroplated on the impression forming electroformed dies. These metals usually have high strength and abrasion resistance. Copper and silver are the commonly used metals; however, Bismuth, lead, etc. have also been used.

   The anode is a bar of pure metal, supplying metal cations continuously. The deposition takes place on the cathode (impression). The impression must be made electrically conducting and it acts like cathode.

   a. **Copper plating:** Copper is usually used with impressions of impression com-pound or addition silicone rubber base material.

   The cavity surface is either coated with colloidal metal or graphite to make it electroconductive.

   Very low amperage is used at the start of electroplating, otherwise the initial deposit of copper is granulated, which may spoil the die. After the entire cavity surface is coated with copper, the amperage may be stepped up to accele-rate the electroforming.

   Plating is allowed to proceed for 12–15 hours. After electroforming, the electro-forming solution is washed off. Acrylic resin or dental stone can be poured.

   b. **Silver plating:** Silver is used with poly-sulfide, polyether and silicone rubber base materials.

   The surface of the impression is metallized with a fine silver powder. A silver cyanide bath is preferred. The reliability of silver cyanide bath is better and also

polysulfide is more dimensionally stable in the alkaline cyanide bath.

An anode of pure silver at least twice the area to be plated is used. Electroplating is carried out for approximately 10 hours. Handling of silver plating solution should be carried out with care since the solution is poisonous.

3. **Amalgam dies:** Conventional amalgam as used for restorations is also used to make dies.

   In case of amalgam dies, the die should be lubricated with oil prior to fabrication of the wax pattern. After the inlay is tried on the amalgam die, it must be pickled to remove any traces of amalgam.

4. **Epoxy resin dies:** The routinely used epoxy resin material is mixed in vacuum and then poured into the impression. It is compatible with all impression materials except hydrocolloids. The resin cures in about half an hour at room temperature.

   During this curing it shrinks about 0.02 to 0.6% depending on configuration and bulk of the die, which can be compensated by thermal treatment of the die.

   Epoxy dies are stronger and more abrasion resistant than gypsum dies and also the reproduction of detail is much better than with gypsum dies.

C. PREPARING THE WAX PATTERN

After the preparation of the die, a lubricant is applied to facilitate the withdrawal of the pattern from the die. Various lubricants used are castor oil, machine oil, petroleum jelly, cocoa butter, etc. The time for the application of the lubricant depends upon the wetness of the die; the humid die will take less time and vice versa.

The inlay wax can be poured directly in increments (Fig. 9.13); alternatively, inlay wax is heated over flame and softened by rotating between fingers and pushed into the cavity keeping under pressure for sometime (Fig. 9.14). Vaseline should be applied to the fingers so that wax may not stick.

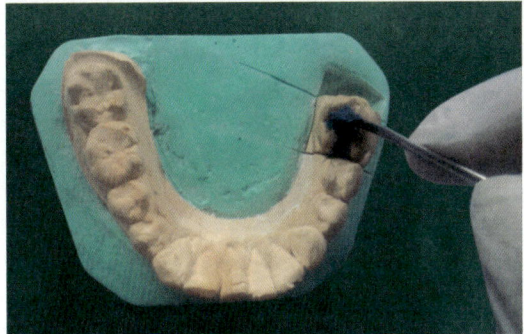

Fig 9.13: *Inlay wax poured in increments*

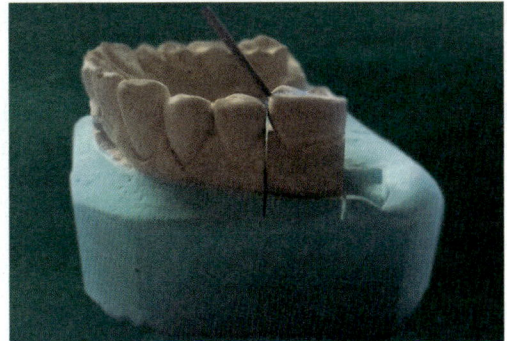

Fig. 9.16: *Attaching sprue former*

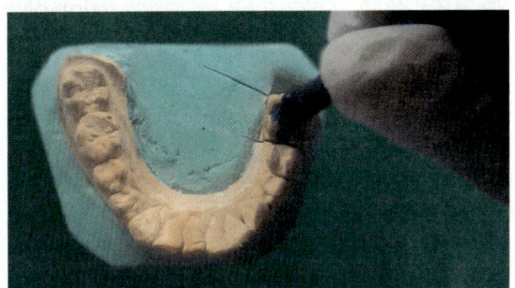

Fig. 9.14: *Inlay wax pushed in bulk*

D. SPRUE ATTACHMENT AND REMOVAL OF PATTERN

The sprue former should be attached to the pattern (Fig. 9.15) while it is still on the tooth to minimize distortion of pattern due to heat and mechanical induction of stresses. The sprue former should be attached to the bulkiest part of the wax pattern (Figs 9.16 and 9.18).

Generally, the sprue former is attached in a position so that the molten metal will reach

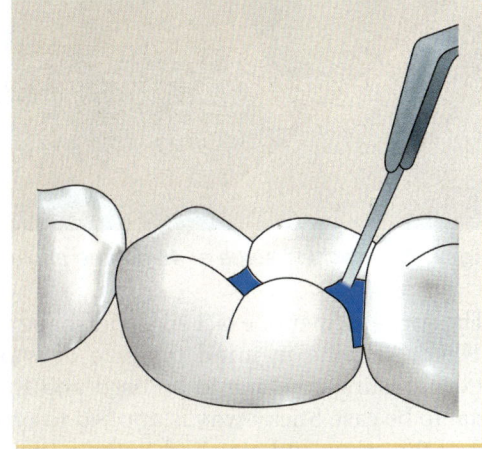

Fig. 9.17: *Angle of sprue former*

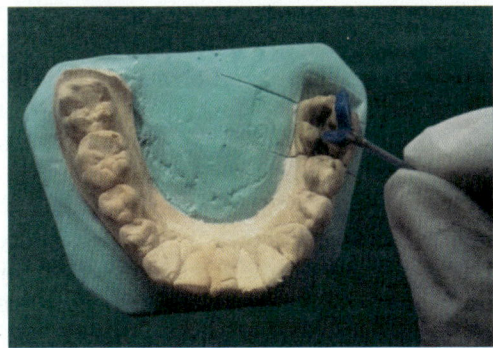

Fig 9.18: *Appropriate area for sprue attachment*

the mold areas farthest from the attachment of the sprue former at the same time. Further, the sprue formers should be attached to the least anatomical area of the wax pattern.

It should not be attached at right angle to a broad surface because the melt may impinge

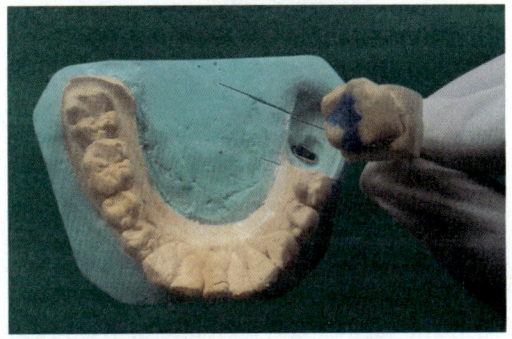

Fig. 9.15: *Prepared pattern*

the mold surface and produce a so-called 'hot spot' producing suck back porosity.

An angle of 45° is usually adequate (Figs 9.17 and 9.19). The sprue former should be directed away from any thin or delicate parts of the pattern, since molten metal may abrade or fracture investment in this area and result in casting failure.

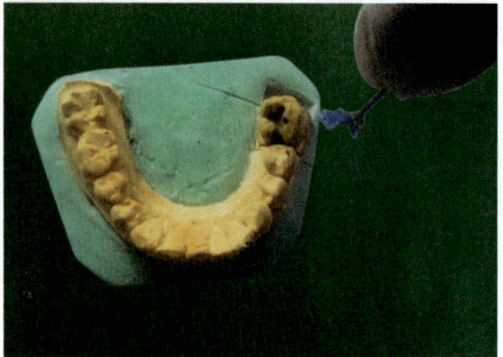

Fig. 9.19: *Attaching sprue at 45 degree angle*

The sprue former of exact size and shape is selected, keeping in mind the size of wax pattern, casting machine to be used and the metal to be cast. Sticky wax is applied to one end of the sprue and attached to the pattern site. A little wax can be added, if need be, at the joining of the sprue and the pattern. After keeping the sprue for 2–3 minutes, trial removal can be carried out. The pattern is to be removed without distortion along the direction of cavity walls. Alternatively, indirect procedure can be used. A copper staple or a 24 gauge twisted brass wire is inserted into the occlusal part of the pattern. For MOD patterns, the prongs of the wire are placed near the marginal ridges and for disto-occlusal or mesio-occlusal patterns, the prongs are inserted at an angle of 45° near the marginal ridge. Using the staple, the pattern is lifted out of the cavity with a direct pull parallel to the cavity walls (Figs 9.20 and 9.21). The sprue is then inserted into the wax pattern and the staple removed by holding it with warm pliers to melt the wax holding the staple. The contact area is built, if need be, using low fusing waxes (Fig. 9.22).

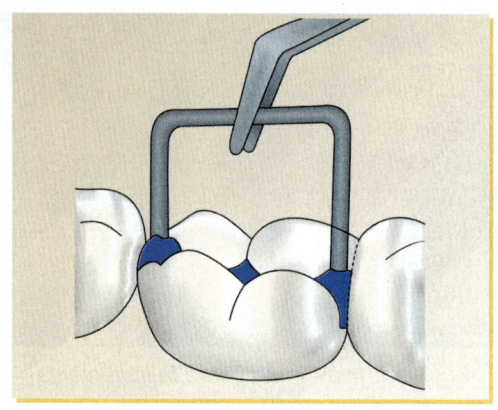

Fig. 9.20: *Putting staple for removing the pattern*

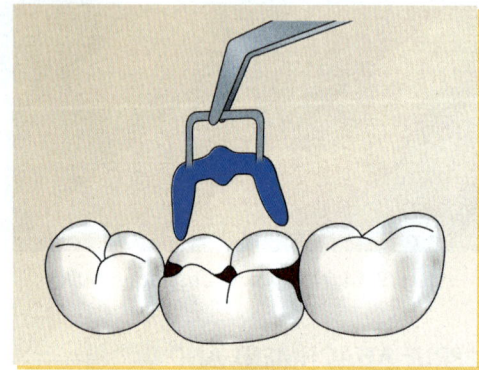

Fig. 9.21: *MOD pattern removed*

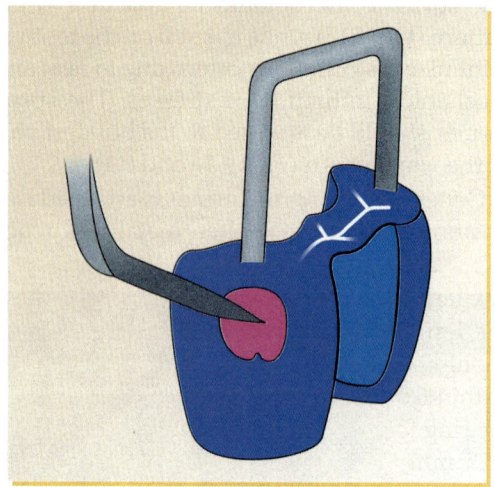

Fig. 9.22: *Building contact area*

Sprue Former Material

The sprue former can be made of wax, resin or metal.

Wax and resin sprue formers have the advantage of being burnable and so do not need to be mechanically removed. However, wax sprue formers lack rigidity.

Metal sprue formers can be solid or hollow. Hollow sprue formers are preferred since they hold less heat than a solid sprue former and so will cause less heat transfer to wax pattern resulting in less distortion. Also their retention to the wax pattern is better. To further improve retention and reduce thermal conductivity, the sprue former can be filled with sticky wax.

The metal sprue former must be mechanically removed prior to burnout. This could cause investment to loosen from the walls. To avoid this, metal sprue formers are uniformly coated with wax.

Sprue Former Diameter

The diameter of the sprue former will depend on the size of the wax pattern, the quality of casting machine, and the ring, which is used to form the mold.

The diameter of the sprue is the most important factor in determining the speed with which the molten metal enters and fills the mold.

Preferably the diameter of the sprue former should not be more than 1/4th of the total area of the wax pattern. Alternatively, it must equal to the size of the thickest part of the wax pattern. If diameter of sprue former is more than wax pattern it leads to distortion. On the contrary, if the diameter of sprue former is less than the wax pattern suck-back porosity might result.

Sprue Former Length

The length of the sprue former depends upon the length of the casting ring. The length should be adjusted so that the wax pattern is within 6.5 mm (1/4 inch) of the open end of the ring for gypsum-bonded investments and 3.25 mm (1/8 inch) for phosphate bonded investments (Fig. 9.24). If the pattern is too close to the end of the ring, the molten alloy may blast through the investment during casting; if it is too far away, gases may not escape rapidly enough to allow metal to fill the mold space.

The sprue former should not be too long such that the gold alloy begins to solidify in the sprue and causes porosity in the casting. In any case, the length of sprue former must not exceed 6–8 mm.

Reservoir

In case, the diameter of the sprue is smaller than the average cross-sectional area of the pattern, a reservoir is attached with the sprue as near as possible to the pattern-sprue junction (Figs 9.23 and 9.24). The diameter of the reservoir should be more than the average cross-sectional area of the pattern. The rationale of adding reservoir to sprue is to provide molten metal to prevent localized shrinkage porosity.

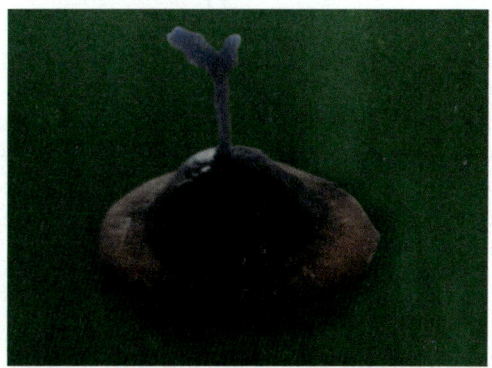

Fig 9.23: *Pattern and the sprue*

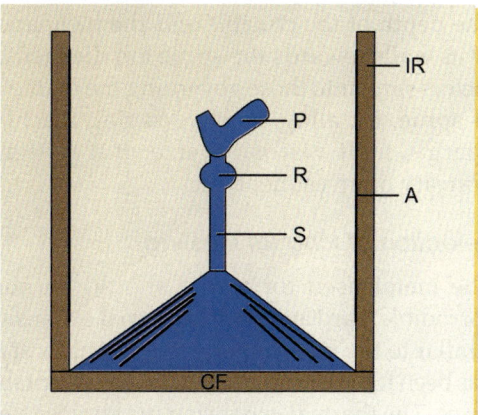

Fig. 9.24: *Pattern, ring and cone CF: crucible former IR: investment ring; A: asbestos lining; P: pattern; R: reservoir; S: sprue*

Principles of Sprue Former	
1. Sprue former length	– Depends on casting ring, such that pattern is within 6 mm of the trailing end
2. Sprue former diameter	– Equal to thickest part of wax patten
3. Sprue former attachment	– Generally flared for gold alloy – May be direct or indirect (reservoir)
4. Sprue former material and type	– May be of wax, plastic or metal – May be hollow or solid
5. Sprue former location/position	– Ideal location is point of greatest bulk in the pattern to avoid distorting thin areas
6. Sprue former direction	– Should be attached 45° to proximal area

When molten metal strikes against the mold wall at 90 degree angle and if the mold-metal temperature differential is more, it creates a hot-spot, the molten metal in this area will solidify last, leading to localized shrinkage porosity, if there is no continuous supply of molten metal. The reservoir provides the molten metal to compensate for this localized shrinkage porosity at the casting-sprue junction.

If we use a sprue former, the diameter of which is greater than the diameter of the cross-sectional area of the pattern, there is no need for providing reservoir. The sprue will itself provide the molten metal.

E. PREPARATION FOR INVESTMENT

Attaching the Sprue to Crucible

The sprue is attached to the crucible in the same way as the sprue is attached to the mold. The depth of the crucible and the inclination of its walls towards the sprue are dictated by factors similar to those governing the diameter of sprue, i.e. alloy density, casting machine energy, melt viscosity, size of a pattern, porosity of investment, etc.

Selection of Ring for Casting

The metal used for a ring should be non-corrodible, hard and with a thermal expansion similar to the investment used. Stainless steel has been found to produce the most acceptable rings. The thermal expansion of stainless steel is 12% at 700°C, which is compatible with the expansion of investments, provided a liner is used.

The dimensions of the ring may vary according to the desire of the operator, but the average dimensions are approximately 29 mm (1 × 1/8 inch) in diameter and 38 mm (1½ inches) in height.

Use of Liner

A resilient liner is placed inside the ring to provide a buffer of pliable material against which the investment can expand to enlarge the mold (Fig. 9.24). If there is no liner present, the investment is in direct contact with the walls of the mold and will not be able to expand outward (because of the resisting action of the walls of ring). In such cases the investment expands towards the centre of the mold thus resulting in distortion of the casting.

Liner Material

Asbestos has been the material of choice to line casting rings; however, its use is restricted because of its cariogenic potential.

Alternatives to asbestos liners have been introduced; these include absorbent cellulose and non-absorbent ceramic materials. Cellulose liners are wetted before use and ceramic liners can be used dry.

The maximum thickness of a liner is 1.0 mm. A 2.0 mm thick liner or two layers of liner can also be used. The liner is cut to fit the inside diameter of the ring with no overlap.

The length of the liner is a controversy.

A few authors are of the view that when a liner is placed 1/8th to 1/4th inch short at each end of the ring, the investment cannot expand laterally at the ends of the ring. In the central portion of the ring it does expand laterally. This expansion may distort the mold.

Many others feel that expansion of the investment is always greater in the unrestricted direction (longitudinal) rather than in the lateral direction (towards the ring itself). Thus it is important to reduce expansion in the longitudinal direction. Liner should be placed 1/8 inch short at the ends to get less distortion of the mold. This becomes more important during cellulose liners which burn before casting is made.

The diagrammatic representation of the ring, crucible former, sprue former, and wax pattern is shown in Fig. 9.24.

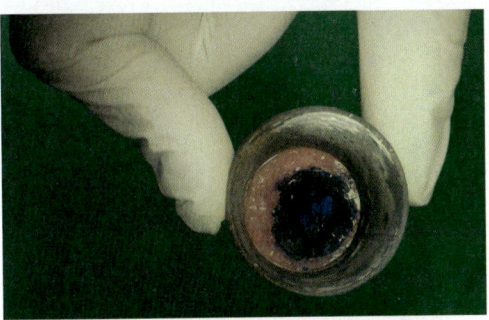

Fig. 9.26: *Investing the pattern*

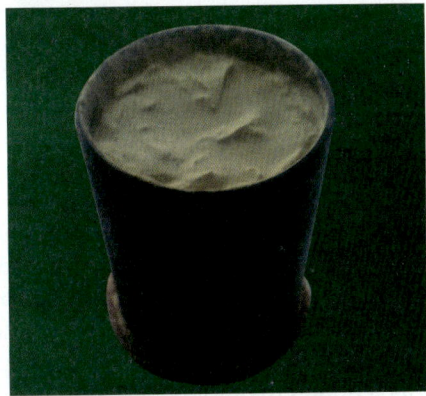

Fig. 9.27: *Investment completed*

Preparing the Wax Pattern for Investment

The wax pattern should be cleaned of any debris or oil before it is positioned in the ring. This will decrease the surface tension and improve the wettability of the wax pattern.

The liquid soap using No.2 paint brush is applied inside and outside the pattern. The soap should be thoroughly rinsed off with water and the pattern is dried with a stream of clean air.

Investing the Pattern

The pattern can be invested either by manual or vacuum investing (Figs 9.25 to 9.27).

Manual Investing

The standardized amount of water and powder are taken in the rubber bowl and mixed with a hand spatula. The mix is placed on a vibrating table and stirred slowly to

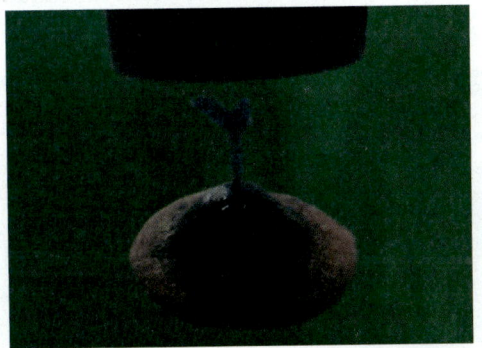

Fig. 9.25: *Investing the pattern*

remove any entrapped air. The investment is then carefully applied to the pattern, using a small sable brush, starting from one side. The investment is allowed to set partially. The rest of the lined ring is then filled with investment.

Vacuum Investing

In this technique, the investment is mixed and the pattern is invested under vacuum. Several types of vacuum investing equipment are available in the market.

Although good results can be obtained both with hand and vacuum investing, the latter technique is preferred because it produces smooth castings.

F. BURNOUT PROCEDURE

The casting ring should be placed in an oven preheated to approximately 900°F (480°C), held at that temperature for 20 minutes, and then the temperature is slowly raised to 1290°F (700°C) and held for 30 minutes (Fig. 9.28).

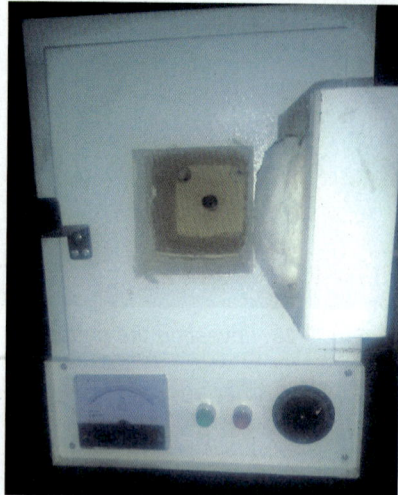

Fig. 9.28: *Heating furnace*

Care should be taken to avoid heating gypsum-bonded investment above 1290°F (700°C). The calcium sulphate is reduced by carbon molecules releasing sulphur dioxide gas at this temperature. The sulphur dioxide gas, thus released may contaminate the gold alloy as it enters the mold.

It is advisable to burnout with the sprue hole facing downward since this will allow the wax to run from the mold and carry investment inclusions out of the mold cavity.

The gold is melted using torch flame using natural gas or a mixture of oxygen and natural gas. For base metals, however, acetylene is used along with oxygen.

G. CASTING MACHINES

Three types of casting machines are available. The variation is in their techniques of pushing gold into the mold.

a. *Air pressure casting machine:* Air, nitrous oxide or even steam is used to push gold.

b. *Vacuum casting machine:* Vacuum is utilized to draw the gold into the mold.

c. *Centrifugal casting machine:* Gold is carried into mold by centrifugal force.

a. Air Pressure Casting Machine

The alloy is melted in the hollow space left by crucible former and then air pressure is applied through a piston, which is pushed downward into contact with the top of the ring, enclosing the molten gold alloy. A pressure of 10–15 psi is usually applied.

b. Vacuum Casting Machine

Vacuum is applied through the base beneath the casting ring and the molten alloy can be drawn into the mold by suction. It cannot work alone in filling the mold, even if gravitational forces are used in driving the melt. Usually the machines are employed that use a combination of gas pressure and a vacuum or centrifugal and gas pressure with the vacuum to create the driving force.

c. Centrifugal Casting Machine

Various designs of the centrifugal casting machines are now available (Fig. 9.29). The machine has a strong spring encased in the base of the casting machine, which can be wound into tension by rotating the arms with the weights at one end and the casting ring at the other. In front of the ring is a separate crucible in which the gold alloy is melted. When the spring is released the two arms rotate rapidly, and the molten metal is forced into the mold by centrifugal force.

Time required to cast gold alloy by centrifugal force depends on the cross-sectional area of the sprue and the number of winds of the machine.

When the size of the sprue is increased, the casting time is reduced. When the number of winds is increased and therefore the force is increased, the casting time is reduced. The cross-sectional area has a greater influence on casting time than does the number of winds of the machine.

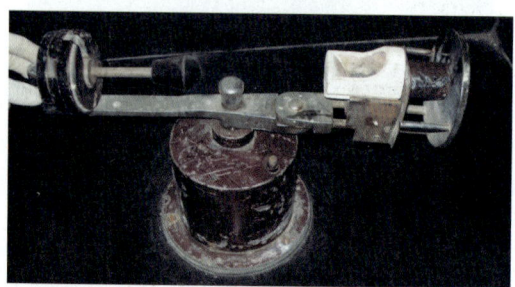

Fig. 9.29: *Centrifugal casting machine*

SUMMARILY

- Centrifugal force is directly proportional to the square of the speed of the machine in revolutions per second.
- Centrifugal force varies directly with the radius of the circular path. Doubling the length of the arm of machine doubles the force.
- Centrifugal force is directly proportional to the weight of the metal directly over the sprue.

Usually centrifugal machines are used; therefore procedure using centrifugal machine is described.

The counter weight of the casting machine is grabbed in the right hand and wound clockwise 2–5 times. The pin is raised from the base so that it rests in front of the crucible assembly, preventing the spring from unwinding. The heated ring from the furnace (Fig. 9.28) is adjusted in the prongs.

Casting alloy is placed in the crucible. Enough bulk of the metal (thirty two times the weight of the pattern) must be used in casting to fill the mold, the sprue and part of the crucible former.

The oxygen gas along with blow-pipe is commonly used to melt the metal. A small multiorifice tip is ideal. The oxygen valve should be opened slowly to prevent sudden high pressure from hitting the regulator and producing high compression heat. Gas is ignited first and extinguished last.

A conical flame about 40 mm long is obtained by adjusting the torch (Fig. 9.30). The reducing part of the flame is used to melt the alloy. The outer, oxidising zone of the flame should not be used since it forms oxides of copper and silver metal used in the alloy.

A small amount of flux should be sprinkled onto the warm metal. Borax, a commonly used flux helps to exclude oxygen from the surface of the alloy and dissolve any oxides that are formed.

Reducing flux, which contains carbon in addition to borax, will also reduce any oxides

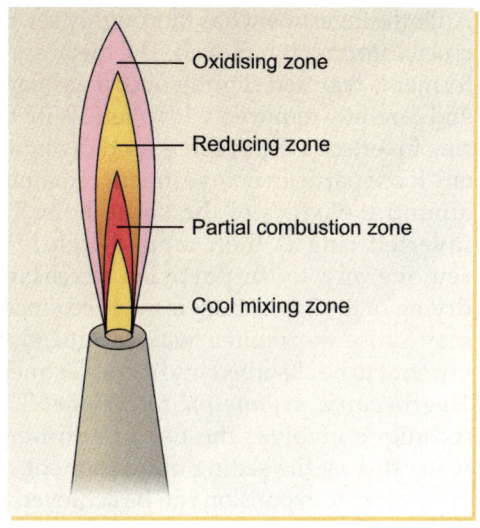

Fig. 9.30: *Parts of flame*

Oxidising zone
Reducing zone
Partial combustion zone
Cool mixing zone

that happen to form. When the reducing zone of the flame is in contact with the metal, the surface will be bright and mirror like. As the alloy melts it first appears spongy, and finally it assumes a spheroidal shape and moves with the flame.

Keeping the flame on the gold, the casting ring is removed from the oven and carefully placed in the cradle of the casting machine.

When the metal is slightly light orange in colour and tends to spin or follows the flame when moved, it is ready to be cast.

Gentle clockwise pressure is applied on the counterweight so that the pin drops. The weight is released allowing the machine to spin. The metal will be thrust into the mold space.

Casting Techniques

The two types of casting techniques are usually used. One using high heat (thermal expansion) and the other using low heat (hygroscopic expansion).

1. *Thermal expansion technique:* The investment is allowed to harden in an open environment. The excess investment is leveled off the surface of the ring before it sets. Scraping at a later stage decreases the porosity of the investment.

After the investment has thoroughly set, the crucible former is removed. The metal sprue former is warmed slightly over a gas flame and carefully removed with pliers. With the ring inverted, a dry brush is used to remove any loose particles of investment remaining around the edges of the sprue hole. The inverted ring is then tapped lightly to remove any loose particles. Excessive drying of the investment is avoided since it may cause the molten wax produced by burnout to be absorbed into the investment.

2. *Hygroscopic expansion technique:* This technique involves the use of additional water during the setting of investment. Hygroscopic expansion can be achieved by two ways:

   i. *Water bath technique:* Immersing the filled casting ring in a water bath at 40–45°C.
   ii. *Controlled water technique:* Addition of a known quantity of water to the exposed surface of unset investment in the casting ring.

The investment is allowed to set for a minimum of 45 minutes. After the investment has set, the investment mold is subjected to burn out and the alloy is cast.

H. CLEANING THE CASTING

After the casting has been completed, the ring is removed and quenched in water as soon as the button emits a dull red glow.

Advantages of quenching are:
- The noble metal alloy is left in an annealed condition for burnishing, polishing, etc.
- When water contacts the investment, it is absorbed into the investment pores. It undergoes immediate vapourizing within the hot mass. Steam in large amounts produces cracking of the investment into small pieces. This simplifies cleaning the casting.

Often the surface of the casting appears dark because of surface oxides and tarnish. The surface film can be removed by pickling. Hydrochloric acid and sulphuric acid is commonly used.

After pickling, the casting should be washed in running water to remove the acid.

CASTING DEFECTS

The various types of casting defects can be:

1. Porosity

The porosity is a major defect commonly encountered in castings. These are further classified as:

a. *Those caused by solidification shrinkage*
   i. *Localized shrinkage porosity:* During solidification of metal in mold, if additional molten metal is not available

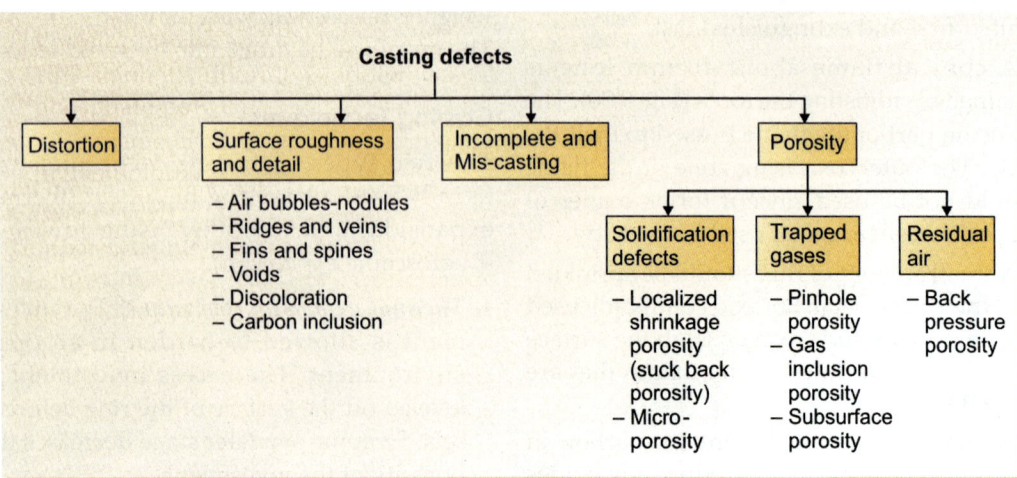

to compensate for shrinkage (usually 1.25%) then porosity occurs.

Mostly it occurs at the sprue casting junction (Fig. 9.31a).

It could also be the result of formation of a hot spot when metal impinges on the mold surface and remains molten while it solidifies at other places.

ii. *Micro porosity:* It occurs due to premature solidification of the metal and is the result of solidification shrinkage.

It occurs due to unduly rapid solidification of the metal or casting temperature is too low.

b. *Porosities caused by gas*

Gases cause either pinhole porosity or gas inclusion porosity.

Both produce spherical defects; the defects in case of gas inclusion porosity are larger.

The metal absorbs gases when it is in molten state. Upon solidification, the absorbed gases are expelled and pinhole porosity results. It can be larger if the reducing zone of the flame is not used.

c. *Subsurface porosity*

The exact reason for this has not been established. It may be due to the simultaneous nucleation of solid grains and gas bubbles at the first moment that the metal freezes at the mold walls.

d. *Back pressure porosity*

Porosity produced due to air entrapped on the inner surface of the casting (Fig. 9.31b). Usually occurs if for some reason gas is not vented from the mold. Mold and casting temperature should not be too low so as to allow metal to solidify rapidly.

2. Incomplete Castings

The causes can be:
- Sprue former too small
- Alloy not hot enough
- Mold too cold
- Ingate obstructed
- Insufficient casting force
- Insufficient gold

3. Rounded Margins

The causes can be:
- Incomplete burnout of wax pattern
- Insufficient heating of alloy before casting
- Improper diameter/length of sprue restricts flow of alloy into the mold. The metal freezes before margins are complete.

4. Pits in Casting

The causes can be:
- Debris in mold
- Dirty wax
- Loose debris in crucible
- Mold temperature too hot

5. Distortion

The causes can be:
- Distortion of wax pattern
- Due to uneven movement of the walls of the pattern when the investment is setting. The gingival margins are forced apart by the mold expansion, whereas the solid occlusal bar of wax resists expansion during the early stage of setting.

6. Surface Roughness, Irregularities

The causes can be:
- Air bubbles on the pattern
- Water films causing ridges and veins on the surface
- Too rapid heating resulting in fins or spines
- Under-heating causing incomplete elimination of wax

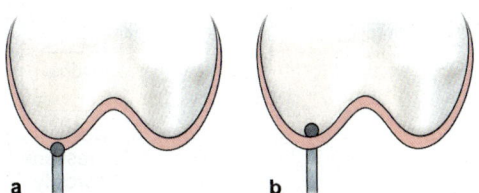

a
Sprue casting
junction
Suck back porosity

b
Inner surface
of casting
Back pressure porosity

Fig 9.31: *Porosity*

- Inappropriate water-powder ratio
- Prolonged heating
- Temperature of alloy too high
- Casting pressure too high
- Foreign bodies
- Impact of molten alloy
- Pattern position

7. Discoloration

The causes can be:
- Sulphur contamination of casting causing black castings
- Contamination with copper during pickling
- Contamination with mercury

The fabrication of cast inlays can be summarized as follows:

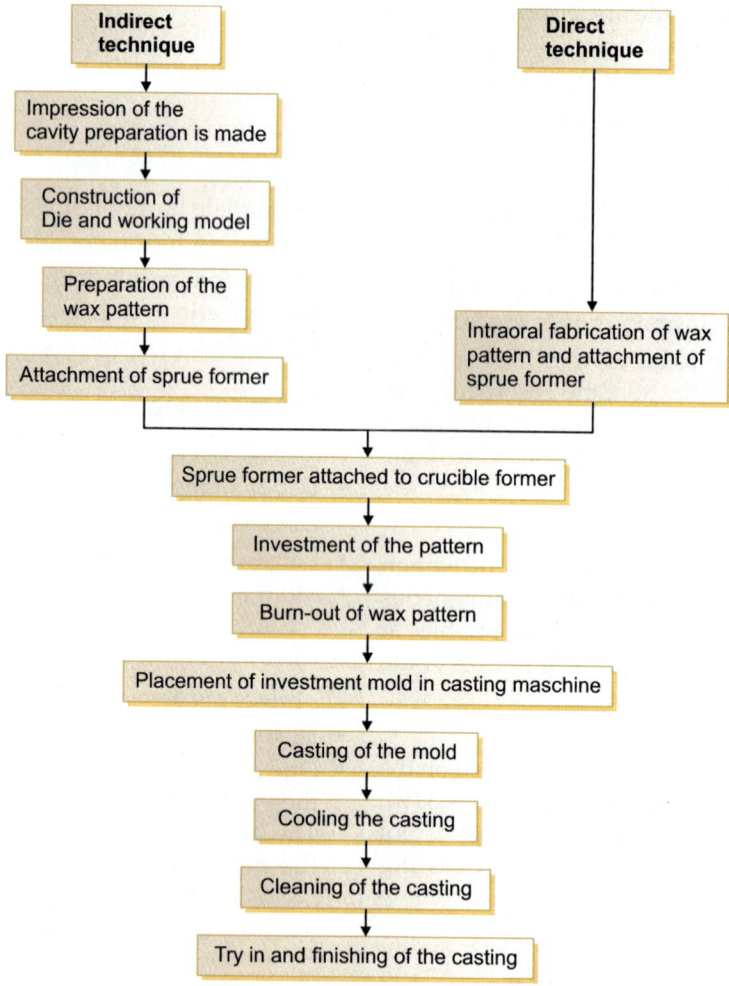

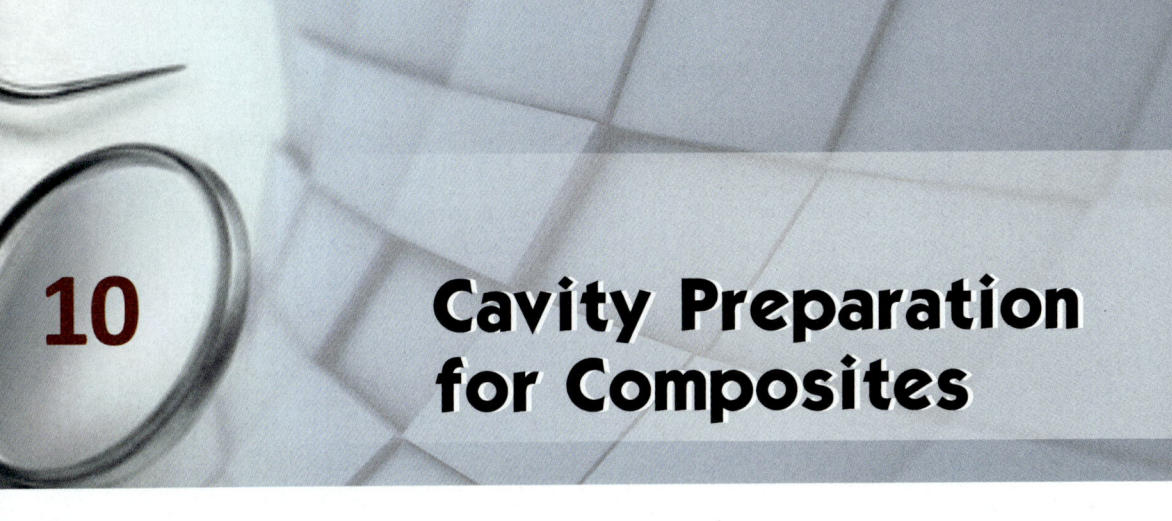

10

Cavity Preparation for Composites

The composite is the most used and abused material these days. The composite restorations, no doubt esthetically pleasing, need extra care during their manipulation. A brief knowledge of composite as a material is important before we proceed with cavity preparation.

The accepted definition of composite is *'Composite material is a compound of two or more distinctly different materials with properties that are superior to or intermediate to those of the individual constituent'.*

COMPOSITION

The composition varies with one brand to another, since plenty of brands are available.

The basic components of composites are:

a. Resin matrix
b. Fillers
c. Coupling agents
d. Coloring agent

a. Resin Matrix

Bisphenol glycidyl methacrylate (BisGMA) was the early resin matrix used. The less viscous varieties such as UDMA (urethane dimethacrylate) and TEGDMA (triethylene glycol dimethacrylate) were introduced later.

b. Fillers

Filler particles made of quartz, silica, trical P, zirconium dioxide, yttrium trifluoride and ytterbium trifluoride have been used in various composites.

Addition of fillers to the resin matrix provides:
- Strength
- Rigidity
- Hardness
- Increase in modulus of elasticity
- Decrease in coefficient of thermal expansion
- Decrease in polymerization shrinkage

The size of the filler particles varies in different composites depending upon the requirements and needs. To ensure acceptable esthetics of composites, the translucency of the filler must be similar to tooth structure.

c. Coupling Agents

Coupling agents are used to bind filler particles to the resin matrix. These agents also provide hydrolytic stability by preventing the water from penetrating along the filler resin interface.

Organic silanes such as γ-methacryloxy-propyltrimethoxysilane are the most commonly used coupling agents.

d. Coloring Agents

Mostly aluminium oxide and titanium dioxide in 0.001–0.007% by wt. are used as coloring agents.

The shade, translucency and opacity should simulate enamel and dentin. The common shades range from yellow to gray.

Difference between chemically cured and light cured composites	
Chemically cured	*Light cured*
• Polymerization is central	• Polymerization is peripheral
• Curing is in one phase	• Curing is in increments
• Sets within 45 seconds	• Sets only after light activation
• No time for manipulation	• Plenty of time for manipulation
• More wastage	• Less wastage
• Not properly finished	• Take better finish

Difference between UV light and visible light used for curing composites	
UV light	*Visible light*
• It works at 360–400 nm	• Light range is 400–480 nm
• Intensity falls with time	• Intensity remains the same
• Injurious to operator's and patient's eyes	• Not injurious
• Greater depth cannot be cured	• Greater depth can be cured

ADVANCES IN COMPOSITES

i. Flowable Composites

Flowable composites were launched to improve upon the handling characteristics of existing composites by decreasing their filler content to 20–25%. These materials have the following features:

Application areas for flowable composites
• Used as filling materials in low stress areas.
• Because of the higher flow, they are useful in areas of difficult access.
• Useful for repairing porcelain.
• Resurfacing worn composite.
• Cementing agents for porcelain restorations.

ii. Packable/Condensable Composites

These composites are based on the concept, called the PRIMM (polymer rigid inorganic matrix material). This system consists of a resin and a ceramic component.

The consistency of PRIMM based composites is similar to that of a freshly triturated mass of silver amalgam, which makes the handling and manipulation much easier.

Packable composites present improved properties over conventional ones, like:
• Increased flexural modulus

• Increased resistance to wear
• Higher depth of cure
• Reduced polymerization shrinkage
• Non-stickiness so that the material can be packed or condensed like dental amalgam.

iii. Antibacterial Composites

Antibacterial composites were introduced with an idea to reduce plaque accumulation over composite resins.

Various agents such as chlorhexidine and MDPB have been tried. Methacryloxydodecyl pyridinium bromide has shown promising results.

iv. Expanding Matrix Resin for Composites

Composite resins that expand slightly during polymerization are desirable. Addition of spiro-orthocarbonates (SOCs) which expand on polymerization will be beneficial. These agents exhibited less shrinkage than the conventional resins but still shrinkage could not be completely eliminated.

v. Bioactive Composites

Calcium phosphate and its modified varieties are being used as filler in recent composites.

These composites serve as bioactive liners and bases to enhance the re-mineralization. These are also referred to as 'Smart Composite'.

Before restoring any lesion with composites, certain factors should be kept in mind.

The factors influencing composite restoration are:

- *Age of the patient:* In very young age, mostly during rampant caries stage, the composite restorations are avoided.
- *Caries index of the patient:* In higher caries index patients, composites are not preferred.
- *Abnormal occlusal contacts and stresses:* Though with the introduction of ceramic filler composites, the problem of stress bearing is improved; yet composites are avoided in such areas.
- Composites are not preferred in areas which cannot be isolated properly.
- Composites are not a material of choice for patients who do not understand the importance of oral hygiene.

Cavity Preparation

There is always a difference of opinion regarding principles of cavity preparation. Certain authors follow conventional GV. Black formulas, while others are of the view that specific width, depth, etc. is not required in composites.

a. *Conventional cavity preparation:* This type of cavity preparation follows: Black's principles of cavity preparation. The outline form includes extension of susceptible lesions, proper uniform depth and the external walls are in accordance with enamel rods. Whether bevel is to be given or not depends upon the following factors.
  - Surface area required for etching
  - Color matching is required or not
  - Area prone to stresses
  - Caries index of the patient

  Bevels are usually recommended on labial surfaces of anterior teeth so as to merge the colour of the composite and the enamel. Lingual bevels can be avoided since colour merging is not of paramount importance. Similarly in class V cavities, bevels are given only on occlusal walls and the gingival walls are spared. In posterior restorations, bevels are not indicated since the thin layers of composite might get chipped off under stresses leading to marginal gaps, sensitivity, etc.

b. *Modified cavity preparation:* Modified cavity preparation does not follow Black's principles and does not have specific width, depth, extension and enamel margins. The retention part is totally dependent upon the etched enamel and bonding. The cavity preparation is usually kept in enamel, if otherwise dictated by the lesion. The individual pits are restored separately. This type of cavity preparation conserves the tooth structure. No definite walls and line angles are visible and usually appear saucer shaped.

Class I Cavity Preparation

The outline is planned keeping in mind the features as described earlier (Fig. 10.1). The surface is cleaned with water and air. A small round bur is used to enter into the caries from the deepest or most carious pit. The movement of the bur is kept parallel to the long axis of

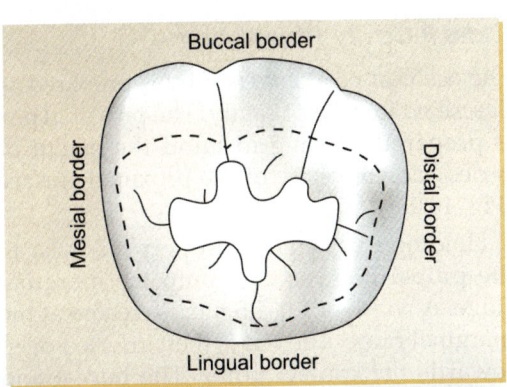

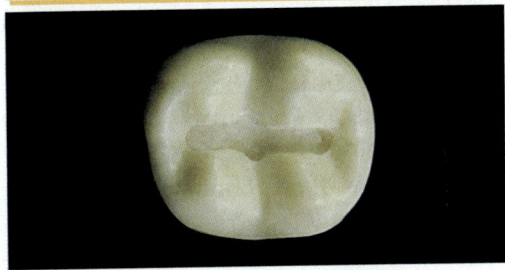

Fig. 10.1: *Class I cavity*

the tooth crown. The depth is kept inside the dentinoenamel junction. The uniformity in the depth can be achieved using flat fissure bur of appropriate size. The depth of the cavity can be kept only in enamel, but for better retention and function, extension into dentin is advisable.

The buccolingual width of the cavity is kept as small as possible, only otherwise dictated by caries. The usual width is 1/4th of the intercuspal distance.

The cavity walls and the floor may not be kept perpendicular and parallel. In deeper cavities, a base of light cure calcium hydroxide or glass-ionomer cement is indicated.

The cavosurface margins are kept at right angle to the cavity walls. No bevel is given. The butt joint preparation minimizes marginal breakdown and ditching of the composites. However, it may lead to marginal staining.

The pits and fissures on the occlusal two-third of the buccal and lingual surfaces of posterior teeth and lingual pits of anterior teeth can be restored with composites in a similar way. Butt joint preparation is preferred. However, a short bevel can be given for merging the colour of composites.

Class II Cavity Preparation

The occlusal part of the cavity is prepared as described for Class I cavity. The proximal box is prepared keeping in mind the extent of caries and convexity of the proximal surface (Fig. 10.2).

Holding a flat fissure bur perpendicular to the pulpal floor, extend onto the marginal ridge. A width of 1.0–1.5 mm is created at the marginal ridge. The bur is then inserted deep towards the contact point. The buccal and lingual walls of the proximal box are kept slightly away from the contact area. These might not be in self-cleansing areas. The gingival wall is kept in enamel without injuring the underlying gingiva.

In case of class II preparation for composites, certain modifications have been suggested.

i. Only proximal box is prepared and the occlusal part is not involved.

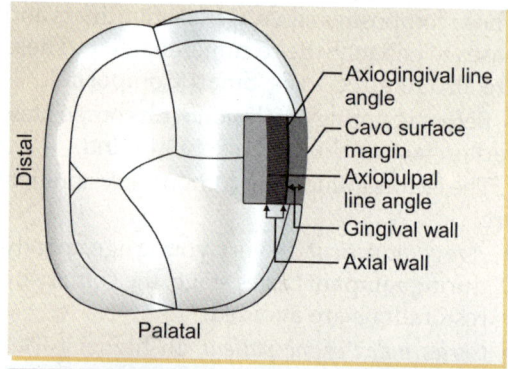

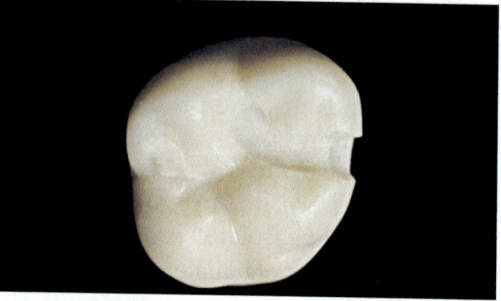

Fig. 10.2: *Class II cavity*

ii. Box only preparation with retentive grooves.
iii. Proximal box preparation with unsupported proximal enamel.

Class III Cavity Preparation

The outline of the cavity depends upon the extent of the lesion proximally and/or labially and lingually. The cavity preparation should always be started from lingual side; in rare instances, labial approach is preferred (Fig. 10.3).

The lingual approach preserves the labial enamel, thereby esthetics of the patient. However, labial approach is indicated in:

• When labial enamel is involved
• Malaligned teeth where lingual approach is difficult
• Rotated teeth where lingual side is hidden

In case labial approach is followed, beveling at the labial enamel wall is indicated to merge the colour of the restoration with the enamel.

The cavity preparation is started using no.1/2 round bur and piercing through the lingual marginal ridge of the concerned side. The direction of the bur is maintained

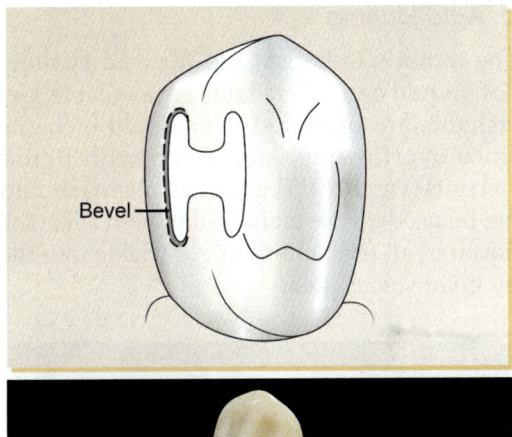

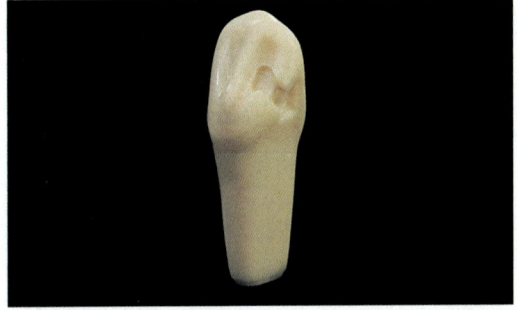

Fig. 10.3: *Class III cavity*

perpendicular to the lingual surface of the tooth, moving the bur 0.5 mm inside the dentinoenamel junction.

The small fissure bur is extended incisially and gingivally creating incisal and gingival walls. The labial enamel is left intact as far as possible. The walls are kept at 90° with the cavosurface margins and bevels are not given. Such a preparation does not have lingual wall. The isthmus between lingual and proximal axial walls should also be kept minimum, preferably not exceeding 1.0 mm.

If facial approach is utilized, then the outline form varies slightly. The small round bur is pierced through the carious lesion maintaining the bur perpendicular to labial surface. Then with small fissure bur, gingival and incisal extensions are given. The cavity preparation is similar to the one described earlier with lingual approach, only difference is that a bevel is to be given on labial cavosurface margin.

The depth of the axial wall should be 0.5 to 1.0 mm. The depth is more incisally and as we move gingivally the depth is decreased.

Final finishing and shaping of the enamel is carried out using hand instruments.

A base of light cure calcium hydroxide or light cure glass-ionomer can be given if indicated.

Class V Cavity Preparation

Restoration of cervical lesions with one surface extending to root or cementum is a common feature. With the advancing age, consequently the recession, the prevalence of cervical erosion and abrasion defects increases. Though glass-ionomer is a preferred choice on such lesions, composites can also be given. In routine patient, composite is preferred because of esthetics.

The outline form is dictated by the extent of the lesion at these sites (Fig. 10.4). The caries or the abrasive/erosive lesion can extend to the cementum or can be totally in cementum. A fissure bur of appropriate size is used to enter the center of the lesion. The bur is kept perpendicular to the axis of the tooth and maintaining the pulpal depth of 0.5 mm below dentinoenamel junction, the bur is moved mesially and distally. The total depth from enamel is 1.0 mm and for cementum is 0.75 to 1.0 mm. The mesial/distal extension is kept within the line angles of the tooth. The gingival wall is contoured according to the cemento-enamel junction and the occlusal wall is more or less straight or slightly curved. The axial wall contour follows the pulp chamber or the outer surface of the tooth.

All the four walls of the cavity, i.e. mesial, distal, occlusal and gingival are kept diverging outwards. The gingival wall, however, is kept straight if it falls in cementum. A short bevel is given on the occlusal wall so as to have better merging of the composite resin with the tooth.

The occlusogingival width of the cavity is kept as minimum as possible unless dictated by caries.

The walls are finished with the help of hand instruments. The cavosurface margin of all the walls is kept at 90° except the occlusal wall where a bevel is placed.

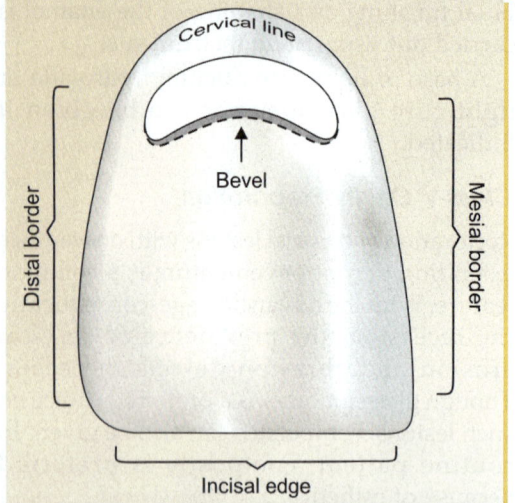

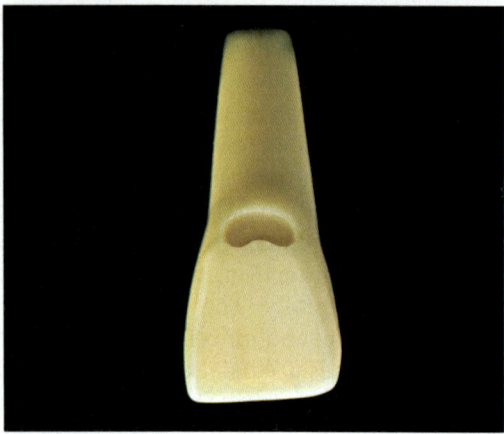

Fig. 10.4: *Class V cavity*

Placement of Composites

The step-wise procedure for composites restorations is as follows:

a. Pulp Protection

After completion of the cavity preparation, the depth of the cavity is evaluated. In case where the depth is more, measures for pulp protection should be undertaken. Calcium hydroxide and glass-ionomers are preferred bases under the composite restorations. Zinc oxide eugenol is contraindicated since it hinders with polymerization of methacrylate group of composite resins. Light cure calcium hydroxide, and glass-ionomers are preferred since over these surfaces, etching is not required.

b. Acid Etching

The tooth is to be isolated for acid etching. Both liquid and gel etchants are available. Gel etchants are preferred over liquid etchants since overflowing is common with liquid etchants (Fig. 10.5). The liquid etchants should not be used on the mandibular teeth since the liquid in all probability might trickle into the gingival sulcus area.

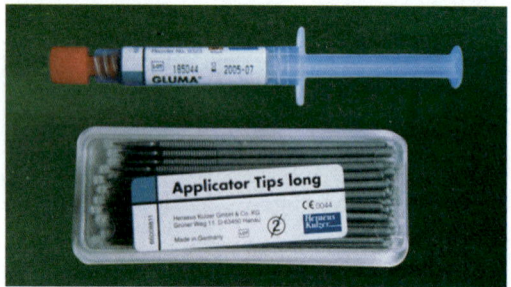

Fig. 10.5: *Etchant and applicator*

The liquid can be applied with cotton pellet or brush. The liquid is gently placed over the surface and should not be rubbed.

The gel etchants can be applied over the surface with the help of plastic instrument, brush or directly applied with the fine needle provided with the syringe. The syringe and needle system is efficient in applying the etchant on the selected surfaces. Care should be exercised not to etch the adjacent teeth and not let the etchant touch the gingival tissues.

After the stipulated time usually 5–10 seconds, the etchant is washed thoroughly. Care should be taken not to leave any residual acid on the cavity walls. The area is dried with oil free air preferably from chip syringe. Compressed air should be avoided as it may injure the enamel tags.

The etched enamel will appear clean, white and frosted. Do not touch the etched surface with any instrument, cotton or hand. In case saliva or gingival fluid escapes isolation and touches the cavity preparation, repeat the procedure again until completely isolated etched surface become available for applying bonding agents.

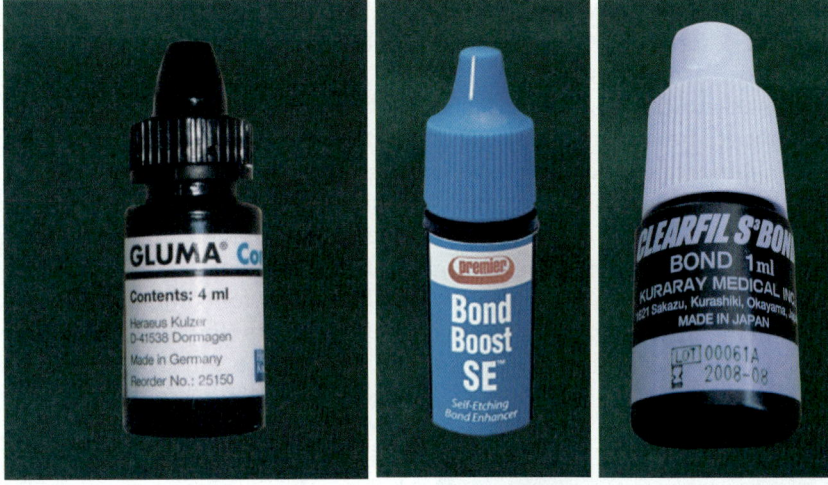

Fig. 10.6: *Bonding agents*

c. Applying Bonding Agent

The bonding agent is applied over the etched surface carefully with the help of brush or the tip designed by manufacturers (Fig. 10.6). One coat of bonding agent is sufficient for enamel; however for dentin, two coats are advised. The first coat is gently rubbed then the second is applied and cured for ten seconds.

Complete isolation should be maintained otherwise if saliva and/or gingival fluid trickle in, the whole process is to be repeated right from etching.

d. Placement of Matrix

Matrices are placed to achieve the proper contact and contour of the tooth. No matrix is required where contours can be controlled, such as class V cavities and cavities on the labial surfaces of anterior teeth, etc.

The matrix should be placed after the etching and bonding steps (Fig. 10.7). In case the matrix is placed before these steps, the application and removal of etchant become difficult.

After placing the matrix, it is stabilized with the help of wedge or impression compound.

Two types of matrices are usually used for composite restorations:

- Metal matrix
- Polyester strips

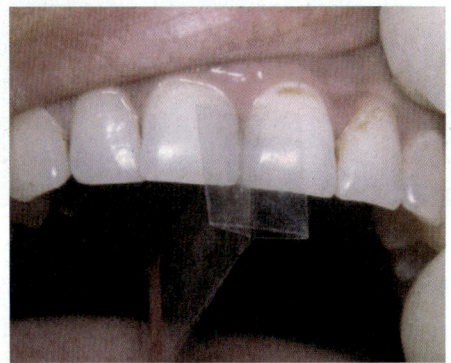

Fig. 10.7: *Applying matrix strips*

The strip or the metal matrix is shaped outside the oral cavity with the help of handle of the mirror or with contouring pliers.

For posterior teeth, relatively thick metal matrix is used since it can resist the condensation pressure with ease and will not give way while packing composite. Transparent matrices, which can reflect light are also used for proximal restorations. In case the transparent matrix is applied, it is exchanged with metal matrix after completing the gingival curing.

e. Restoration

Since most of the composites used these days are light cured, emphasis will be laid on restoration with light cure composites only.

Teflon coated instruments are preferred to pick and insert the composites. Stainless steel instrument should not be used since the composite will stick to the instrument. The instrument should be kept dry during manipulation. In no case the instrument should be touched with hands or any moist object.

Syringes with flowable composites are available with disposable needles to be applied directly at the surface (Fig. 10.8). Guns with ampules of viscous composites are also available.

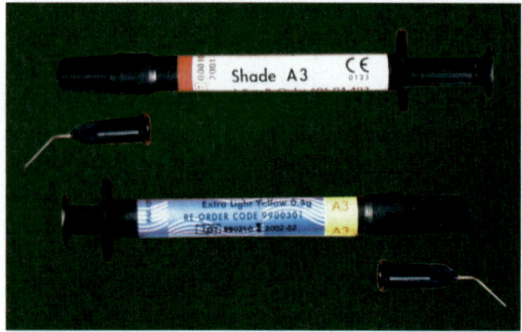

Fig. 10.8: *Flowable composite*

Restoring Class III and Class IV Lesions

After etching, bonding and stabilizing the matrix, the composite in small increment is placed first at the gingival wall. Whether the approach of cavity preparation is labial or lingual, the gingival wall is first to be restored. The first increment should be kept small; approximately 1.0 mm thick and the subsequent increments of 1.0–1.5 mm thickness can be applied over the first. Each increment is cured for 20 seconds and final one cured for 40 seconds to one minute. If lingual approach is utilized, curing is preferred from labial aspect and vice versa in case labial approach is followed. Finally, the composite should be cured from all the surfaces.

Blending of shades in class III and class IV composites is very important. The extent of the lesion and the labial involvement will dictate the amount of blending we use. The darker shade is given at the cervical area followed by less darker in middle and lighter at the incisal areas.

Restoring Class I and Class II Lesions

After the process of etching and bonding is completed, the matrix is stabilized for class II lesions. The volume of the cavity will dictate the operator regarding number and locations of the increments.

The cavity for composite is always restored in increments (Fig. 10.9). The increments can be given in a variety of designs, but the thickness of the increment should be kept as small as possible, i.e. not exceeding 1.5 mm at a time. Each increment is cured for 20 seconds before placing the next over it. Recently few authors are of the view that partial curing of these increments would lead to better adaptation of each increment. This phenomenon is known as 'soft start polymerization' in which the initial increments are cured for 10 seconds. The layers can be placed horizontally one above the other or vertically one joining the other. Alternatively one flat increment at the base and two oblique on the side walls can be given.

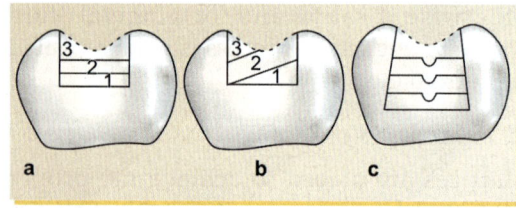

Fig. 10.9a to c: *Different types of increments for restoring composite*

Precaution during Composite Restorations

Composite restorations are very technique sensitive; therefore utmost care is necessary before, during and after their manipulation.

The precautionary measures should be taken at every step; however, the following steps need extra care for the success of composite restorations:

  i. *Complete excavation of caries:* During cavity preparation, the caries should be thoroughly removed. The left over caries hinders with the bonding mechanism.

ii. *Proper etching and removal of residual acid from the enamel tags:* Proper concentration of acid along with proper etching time is mandatory to achieve the requisite tags. Many a times, the acid is not washed out thoroughly and the residual acid in the tags hinders with the bonding, subsequently failure of the restoration.

iii. *Application of bonding agent:* Bonding agent is to be applied gently and uniformly all around the cavity walls. The cavity walls are not to be touched after the bonding.

iv. *Touch of composite with fingers:* The composite in any case should not be touched with fingers. Always pick and hold the composite with Teflon-coated instruments.

v. *Placement of composites:* The composite is to be placed in increments and each increment should be as small as possible, since the contraction after polymerization leads to gaps at the tooth restoration interface.

vi. The curing of the composite should be from all the sides and for stipulated period. The filter and the bulb vis-à-vis the intensity of the light should be checked off and on to ensure the proper curing.

vii. Composites should be finished and polished thoroughly especially at the beveled areas. The occlusion should be checked before final polishing.

Finishing and Polishing

A surface finish attained with the use of a plastic matrix band is the most desirable finish for resin restorations; however, the need for contouring and removal of excess material, make it difficult to obtain such finish. Hence, it is advisable to contour the unpolymerized composite with hand instruments, so that the need for removal of large amounts of set resin leading to surface damage are minimized. The finishing is difficult in conventional composites owing to the nature of filler contents. Micro-filled composites can be finished and polished to the highest gloss.

Excess composite at the cavosurface margins is scraped away using a scalpel or a sharp gold knife. The use of stainless steel instruments should be avoided, as these tend to leave grey marks on the restoration. For gross contouring and finishing of the concave and comparatively non-accessible areas on the occlusal surface, the alpine stone, 12–30 fluted carbide burs and diamond points are recommended (Fig. 10.10). These are preferably rotated at slow speed. Rotary instruments should always be used with a steam of water and little pressure. In the accessible and convex areas of the occlusal surface, agents such as aluminium oxide, cuttle fish or silicon dioxide coated disks and strips are used in a descending grade of their abrasiveness (Fig. 10.11). These instruments are used at very low speeds. Vaseline or petroleum jelly should be used as lubricant with these disks and strips.

For the proximal surfaces, the matrix is removed and the restoration inspected for any voids or faulty contour. Excess composite is removed with scalpel or thin knife. Finishing is required in the gingival embrasure area to

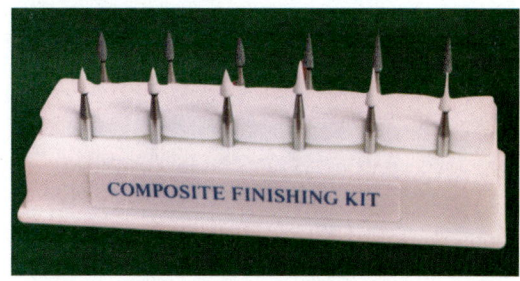

Fig. 10.10: *Finishing kit*

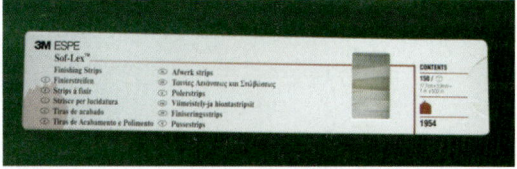

Fig. 10.11: *Finishing strips*

reduce gingival irritation. A very fine abrasive should be used so that the surface inside the restoration is not flattened. Strips are used with short strokes.

For a class V composite restoration, the rotary instruments are preferred. The use of sandpaper disks may damage the gingiva and nick the cementum of the tooth.

The final luster is obtained with polishing pastes that may contain pumice, silica, silicon carbide and zirconium silicate, etc. The paste is made by mixing the abrasive with water or glycerine and carried to the restoration with brushes. White rubber cups are preferred to avoid discoloring the resin and should be rotated slowly with light pressure (Fig. 10.12). After the polishing is completed, air is used to blow away any remaining abrasive particles. Dental floss is used to clean the proximal embrasures of any remaining paste and the restoration finally inspected for any deficiency.

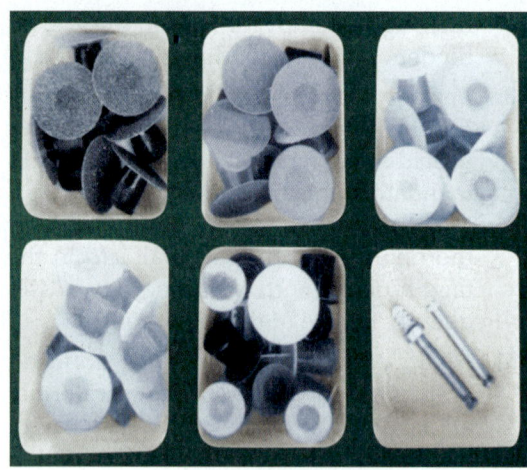

Fig. 10.12: *Polishing kit*

After the final polishing of the composite is completed, a thin layer of glaze may be applied to improve surface smoothness. Glaze is a film of unfilled polymers with a composition similar to the resin matrix.

11 Dental Cements and Varnish

The term cement has been applied traditionally to powder/liquid materials which when mixed to paste consistency, set to form a hard mass. Clinically, cements are used as substitute of dentin and also as luting agents for indirect restorations. A few types of cement are also used to restore the teeth.

The different applications of cements make varying demands for their manipulative properties, working and setting times, resistance to mechanical breakdown and dissolution in oral fluids. Since single type of cement is unlikely to satisfy all these conditions, so specific cements must be selected and developed for specific application.

Usually the cements exhibit acid–base reaction. Some cements show polymerizing reactions. Cements exhibiting both the varieties are also available.

The routinely used cements are:

A. Zinc oxide–eugenol
B. Zinc phosphate cement
C. Polycarboxylate cement
D. Glass-ionomer cement
E. Calcium hydroxide

A. ZINC OXIDE–EUGENOL

Zinc oxide–eugenol is the most widely used temporary restorative material (Fig. 11.1). It offers much better biocompatibility than rest of the dental cements.

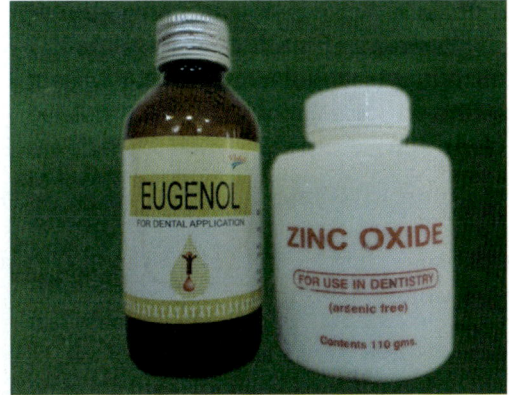

Fig. 11.1: *Zinc oxide–eugenol*

Composition

The composition of conventional zinc oxide–eugenol is:

Ingredients	Weight
Powder	
Zinc oxide	69.0%
White rosin	29.3%
Zinc stearate	1.0%
Zinc acetate	0.7%
Liquid	
Eugenol	85.0%
Olive oil	15.0%

Earlier cements contained 75% zinc oxide and 25% pulverized glass or silica as powder and a liquid component having zinc chloride and a little borax. Later the liquid was replaced with eugenol. Zinc stearate, zinc acetate, magnesium chloride and acetic acid were added, which act as accelerators. Within limits, greater the ratio of zinc oxide to eugenol (powder to liquid), faster is the setting. Water is mandatory to initiate the reaction and it is also a byproduct of the reaction (autocatalytic reaction). This is why the reaction proceeds more rapidly in the humid environment.

$$Zn + H_2O \rightarrow Zn(OH)_2$$
$$Zn(OH)_2 + 2HE \rightarrow ZnE_2 + 2H_2O$$

| Base | Acid | Salt (Zinc eugenolate) |

Types

- Type I — Temporary cementation
- Type II — Permanent cementation
- Type III — Base and temporary restoration
- Type IV — Cavity liners

Properties

- Powder/liquid ratio is 4:1 to 6:1 by weight.
- Setting time is 4 to 10 minutes.
- Compressive strength varies between 14 and 20 MPa.
- Tensile strength is between 0.3 and 2.0 MPa
- Modulus of elasticity is 0.03×10^6 psi

Advantages

- It is a good insulator and sealer of pulp dentin organ.
- It has an antiseptic effect (due to eugenol present in liquid).
- It has a sedative and anti-inflammatory action.
- When inserted into the cavity it has an approximately neutral pH of 7.0 making it one of the least irritating materials.

Drawbacks

- Strength (14–20 MPa) is not sufficient enough to resist forces of mastication.
- Lacks resistance to wear
- High solubility in the oral cavity (0.1–0.2%) as compared to other cements.

To overcome the drawbacks, modified varieties of zinc oxide–eugenol were marketed; some of them are:

i. Resin reinforced zinc oxide–eugenol cements (Fig. 11.2)

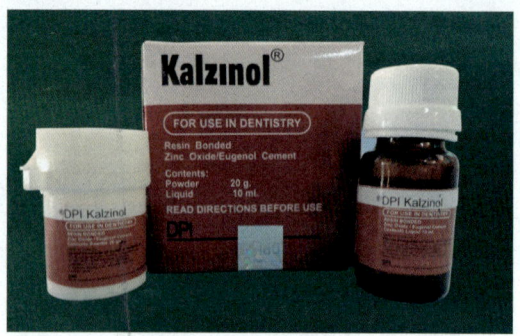

Fig 11.2: *Reinforced ZOE*

Composition

Ingredients	Weight
Powder	
Zinc oxide	80.0%
Zinc methyl-methacrylate	20.0%
Zinc stearate	Traces
Zinc acetate	Traces
Thymol	Traces
Liquid	
Eugenol	85.0%
Olive oil	15.0%

Properties

- Resin increases the strength, homogeneity and smoothness of the mix while it decreases flow and solubility (0.03%).
- Powder/liquid ratio is 4:1
- Setting time is 6–9 minutes
- Compressive strength is 37–40 MPa
- Tensile strength is 4 MPa
- Modulus of elasticity is also improved (0.05×10^6 psi)

ii. Ethoxy benzoate zinc oxide–eugenol cement

Composition

Ingredients	Weight
Powder	
Zinc oxide	70.0%
Alumina/fluid quartz	30.0%
Liquid	
EBA	62.5%
Eugenol	37.5%

Advantages

- Increases compressive (60–80 MPa), tensile (5–8 MPa) and shear strength.
- Decreases solubility (0.05%) and disintegration characteristics.
- In place of eugenol, vanillate ester was added in the liquid to overcome the disadvantages of eugenol.

iii. Cavit

It is a premixed non-eugenol paste used for temporary restorations and cavity bases.

It contains:

- Zinc oxide
- Zinc sulphate
- Calcium sulphate
- Glycol acetate
- Polyvinyl acetate
- Polyvinyl chloride acetate
- Red pigments

B. ZINC PHOSPHATE CEMENT

Zinc phosphate cement is the oldest and time tested cement used in dentistry (Fig. 11.3). It is used both as base and for cementation of indirect restorations. A film thickness of 25 μm makes it preferable cementing medium. The compressive strength of zinc phosphate is equivalent to dentin, therefore preferred as bases under the metallic restorations. However, being exothermic, care is exercised not to use it in deeper cavities. A sub-base is preferred under zinc phosphate cement in deeper cavities (Fig. 11.4).

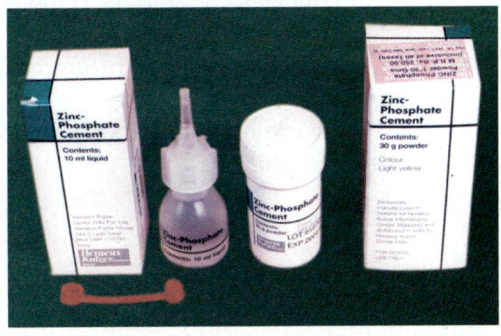

Fig 11.3: *Zinc phosphate cement*

Composition

Ingredients	Weight
Powder	
Zinc oxide	90.2%
Magnesium oxide (MgO)	8.2%
Silicon dioxide (SiO_2)	1.4%
Bismuth trioxide (Bi_2O_3)	0.1%
Barium oxide (BaO)	Traces
Barium sulphate (Ba_2SO_4)	Traces
Calcium oxide (CaO)	Traces
Liquid	
Phosphoric acid (free acid)	38.2%
Phosphoric acid (combined with aluminium and zinc)	16.2%
Aluminium	2.5%
Zinc	7.1%
Water	36.0%

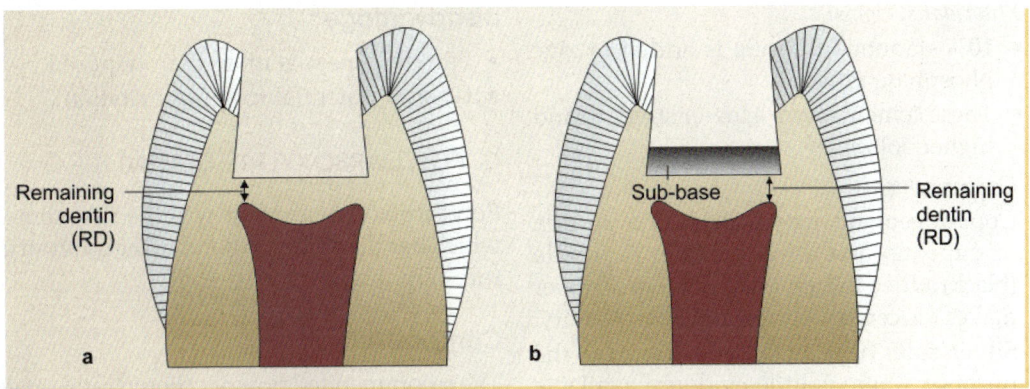

Fig. 11.4a and b: *Base application. (a) Remaining dentin (RD) is less than 1.0 to 1.5 mm, (b) thickness of 0.5 to 0.75 mm sub-base is applied*

Types

Type I : Fine grained for luting
Film thickness should be 25 μm or less
Type II : Medium grained for luting and filling
Film thickness should not be more than 40 μm

Properties

- *Setting time:* 4–7 minutes
- *Powder/liquid ratio:* The more the powder incorporated into liquid, better are the physical properties. Powder/liquid ratio for restorative cement is 2.5:1 and for luting cement is 1.5:1.
- Strength
  - Compressive strength is between 98 and 133 MPa
  - Tensile strength is 5.5 MPa
- It exhibits good thermal and electrical resistance.
- When freshly mixed, cement is highly acidic (pH 1.6), after 24 hours its pH rises to 6 or 7.

Applications

- Commonly used for luting indirect restorations.
- As a base under metallic restorations.
- As a temporary filling material.
- Cementation of orthodontic bands.

Certain modified zinc-phosphate cements are also available. These are:

i. *Fluoridated cements*
- 10% stannous fluoride is added to zinc phosphate powder.
- These cements have a lower strength and higher solubility.

ii. *Copper cements*
Copper cements may consist of a portion of cuprous oxide (red) or cupric oxide (black) added to zinc oxide powder. Copper makes the cement germicidal in oral cavity. Silver salts have also been tried for the purpose. There is little evidence available for any advantage of these cements over conventional cements.

iii. *Zinc silico phosphate cements*
Zinc silico phosphate cement is a combination of zinc phosphate and silicate cement. These are used to cement indirect restorations, especially porcelain (because of their translucency), orthodontic bands and as temporary restorations.

Composition

The powder consists of a combination of silicate glass having 13–25% fluoride and zinc oxide. A small amount of silver may be added to make it germicidal.

The liquid contains:

Phosphoric acid	–	50%
Water	–	45%
Zinc	–	4–9%
Aluminium	–	2%

Properties

- Compressive strength varies between 135 and 175 MPa.
- Tensile strength is 7 MPa
- These materials are more abrasion resistant than zinc phosphate cements.
- Solubility less than zinc phosphate cements.
- Better bonding to tooth structure.
- Fluoride release is evident.
- More translucent than zinc phosphate.
- Mix is highly acidic and pH remains low after setting for prolonged periods of time.

Disadvantage

- Film thickness is more than required.
- Greater potential for pulp irritation.

C. POLYCARBOXYLATE CEMENT

Polycarboxylate cement was the first cement which has the ability to bond to the tooth structure (Fig. 11.5).

Composition

The recommended powder/liquid ratio ranges from 1:1 to 1:2. The higher ratio is for restorative purposes.

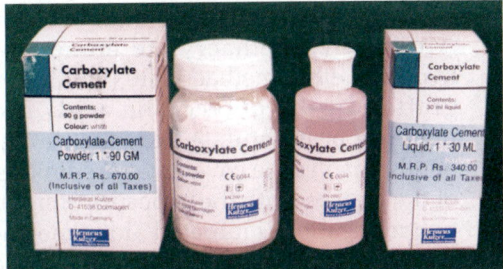

Fig. 11.5: *Zinc polycarboxylate*

Powder	Weight
Zinc oxide	90%
Magnesium oxide	10%
Silica	Traces
Alumina	Traces
Bismuth salts	Traces
Liquid	
Polyacrylic acid	45%
Copolymer of acrylic acid, itaconic acid, maleic acid	2.5%
Tartaric acid	2.5%
Water	50%

Properties

- *Setting time:* It ranges from 6 to 9 minutes at 37° C.
- *Film thickness:* 25 μm.
- *Strength:* Compressive strength is 55–85 MPa; whereas, tensile strength is 8–12 MPa.
- *Bond strength to enamel:* 3.45 – 13.1 MPa
- *Bond strength to dentin:* 2.07 MPa.
- The pH of the liquid is 1.5 which is rapidly neutralized by the powder.

Advantages

- Low level of irritation
- Adhesive to tooth
- Easy manipulation
- Strength, solubility and film thickness are comparable to zinc phosphate.

Disadvantages

- Accurate proportioning is mandatory for optimum properties.
- Lower compressive strength.
- Greater visco-elasticity than zinc phosphate.
- Short working time.

D. GLASS-IONOMER CEMENT

The original glass-ionomer cement is a hybrid formulation of silicate and poly carboxylate cements (Fig. 11.6). The earliest preparation was called 'ASPA' (aluminosilicate polyacrylic acid).

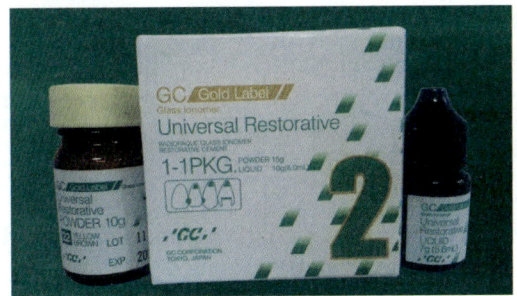

Fig. 11.6: *Glass ionomer cement*

Composition

Powder	Weight
Silica	35–50%
Alumina	20–30%
Aluminium fluoride	1.5–25%
Calcium fluoride	15–20%
Sodium fluoride	3–6%
Aluminium phosphate	4–12%
Lanthanium, strontium, barium	Traces
Liquid	
Polyacrylic acid	45%
Itaconic acid	
Maleic acid	
Tricarboxylic acid	5% (decreases viscosity)
Tartaric acid	Traces (increases working time and decreases setting time)
Water	50% (Hydrates reaction product)

Properties

- Glass-ionomer cement releases fluoride comparable to those released from silicate cement which continues over an extended period.
- Glass-ionomers are relatively biocompatible.
- Mixing time is 30 seconds.

- Working time is 60–90 seconds.
- The recommended power/liquid ratio is 3.5 gm/ml.

Advantages

- Adhesion to enamel and dentin.
- Fluoride release.

Disadvantages

- Main disadvantage is its opaque nature
- Poor strength; hence not considered for posterior restoration.

Certain modified glass-ionomer cements available are:

i. Metal reinforced glass-ionomer cement (Glass Cermet)

Glass-ionomer cement cannot withstand high stresses because it lacks toughness. It can be reinforced by physically incorporating silver alloy powder with glass powder (Fig. 11.7), or by fusing glass powder to silver particles through sintering.

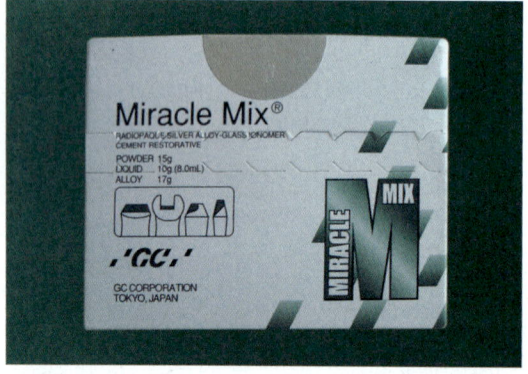

Fig. 11.7: *Miracle Mix*

Drawbacks

- Metallic fillers have little or no influence on mechanical properties of restorative glass-ionomer.
- Both metal-reinforced systems release appreciable amounts of fluoride initially, but the magnitude decreases substantially over time.
- Materials are gray in colour because of metallic phases within them, therefore, they are unsuitable for use in anterior teeth.

ii. Resin modified glass-ionomer cements

A dimethyl methacrylate monomer, hydroxyl ethyl methacrylate (HEMA) is grafted in the polyacrylic acid. The presence of unsaturated carbon–carbon bonds enables the covalent cross-linking of the matrix. With the exposure of light, polymerization is initiated along methacrylate groups. After that the polyacrylic acid reacts with glass particles through acid–base reaction. The main reaction is acid–base reaction. They maintain the ability to bond to hard tooth tissues via the carboxylic group of polyalkenoate component. Fluoride release is also optimal. Fuji II LC is one commercial preparation of resin modified glass-ionomer (Fig. 11.8).

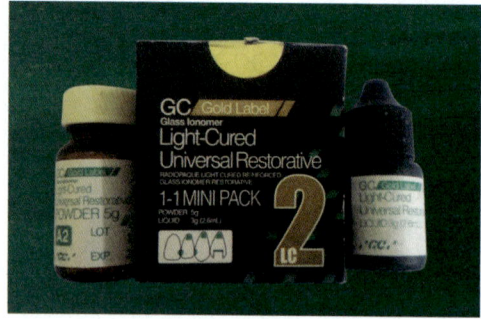

Fig. 11.8: *Light cure GIC*

They are widely used in class V, erosion/abrasion cavities and also in rampant caries. They are well tolerated by the pulp and can be finished and polished properly.

Advantages

- Stronger
- Nearly insoluble
- Fluoride release
- Good radiopacity
- Easy manipulation
- Satisfactory wear resistance
- Better esthetics
- Early resistance to water attack
- Bond strength — excellent
- Minimal or no postoperative sensitivity
- Condensable viscosity
- Light/dual cure setting

- Long working time
- Can be finished and polished immediately after set

Disadvantages

- Polymerization shrinkage due to residual monomer increases chances of microleakage.
- The manipulation is time consuming.

To overcome disadvantage of dual-cure glass-ionomer cements, a third mode of curing is incorporated. The water activated catalyst allows the methacrylate group to get cured in dark. Such type of glass-ionomer cement is referred to as tri-cure glass-ionomer cement.

iii. Compomer

The compomer is a combination of glass-ionomer and composites, providing advantages of both. The properties are similar to that of composites. It also has the ability to release fluoride and it undergoes an acid–base reaction in the presence of saliva. One paste compomer releases less fluoride than conventional or hybrid glass-ionomer cement. The bond strength of compomer to tooth structure is comparable to conventional glass-ionomer cement.

Two varieties of compomer are available having polyacid monomer with or without water. The compomer containing water is self-adhesive; whereas, the one without water is not self-adhesive.

iv. Giomers

Giomers are hybrid restorative materials which employ the use of pre-reacted glass-ionomers. The fluoroalumino glass in these materials is reacted with poly-alkenoic acid in water prior to inclusion into silica filled urethane resin. The acid–base reaction in these materials has already occurred.

Like compomers, giomers are light poly-merized and require bonding system for adhesion to tooth structure. Giomers are available in one-paste form. They are bio-compatible, clinically stable, show excellent aesthetics, smooth surface finish and also have the ability to release fluorides.

E. CALCIUM HYDROXIDE

Calcium hydroxide has long been recognized as a valuable pulp capping material which facilitates the formation of reparative dentine.

Uses

- As sub-base under deep cavities
- As a base, especially under composite restorations
- As an interim restoration

One commercial form of calcium hydroxide is Dycal (Fig.11.9).

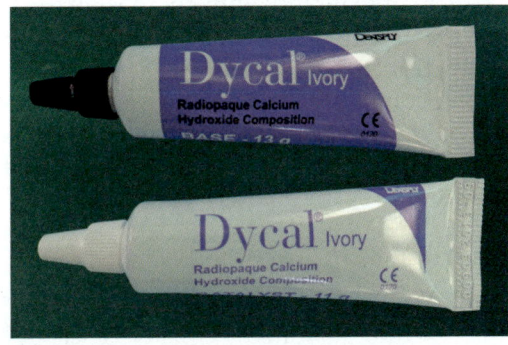

Fig. 11.9: *Dycal*

DYCAL

It consists of two tubes; one tube contains base and the other catalyst.

Base Paste

- Zinc oxide
- Calcium phosphate
- Calcium tungstate
- Iron oxide
- 1,3-butylene glycoldisalicylate

Catalyst Paste

- Calcium hydroxide
- Zinc oxide
- Zinc stearate
- Iron oxide
- N-ethyl p-toluene sulfonamide

Properties

- The base and catalyst are mixed in the ratio of 1:1.

- The setting time is approximately one minute.
- They are quick setting materials.
- Compressive strength after one hour: 10 MPa.
- Tensile strength after one hour: 1.5 MPa.

Advantages

- Improved strength
- Minimal solubility
- Easy manipulation and control over working time
- Rapid hardening in thin layers
- Better compatibility with composites

Over the years, calcium hydroxide has been modified to have better physical properties and biocompatibility. Light-cured calcium hydroxide was introduced which contains resin of composites and light initiators and activators.

Cavity Varnish

Cavity varnish is a solution of one or more resins which when applied onto the prepared cavity walls, evaporates leaving a thin resin film that serves as a barrier between the restoration and dentinal tubules (Fig. 11.10).

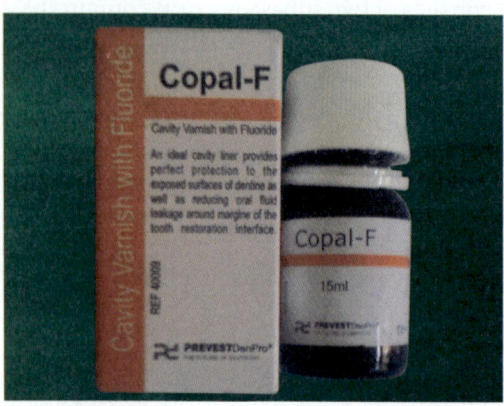

Fig. 11.10: *Cavity varnish*

Indications

- Newly placed amalgam restorations to decrease microleakage, thereby reducing postoperative sensitivity.
- For restoration or base to decrease passage of irritants into freshly cut dentinal tubules.

- In amalgam restorations as it prevents the penetration of corrosion products in dentinal tubules thereby preventing tooth discoloration.
- As surface coating over glass-ionomer restorations to protect them from dehydration.
- As temporary insulator to prevent galvanic currents.

Contraindications

- In composite resins, solvent of varnish softens resin and interferes in polymerization.
- In glass-ionomer cements, varnish eliminates its adhesion potential.
- The therapeutic effect of zinc oxide eugenol and calcium hydroxide is eliminated if varnish is used.

Composition

Natural gum such as copal, resin or synthetic resin dissolved in an organic solvent such as alcohol, acetone or ether. Additives like chlorambutamol, thymol, eugenol and fluorides can be present.

Application

The varnish is applied in thin layers and each layer is dried separately. Usually two coats are considered adequate. More than two coats may cause reduction in mechanical retention.

Properties

- Do not have mechanical strength nor provide thermal insulation
- Film thickness varies between 2 and 40 μm
- Low solubility
- Insoluble in distilled water

Precautions

- To prevent loss of solvent by evaporation, tightly cap the bottle after use.
- Should be applied in thin consistency. Viscous varnish will not wet cavity walls properly.
- Excess of varnish should not be left on margins of restorations as it prevents proper finishing.

12 Preliminary Endodontics

Endodontics is the branch of dentistry which deals with diagnosis, prognosis, treatment and prevention of diseases of pulp and periapical tissues. Basically the word Endodontics is synonymous with root canal treatment. The root canal treatment is divided into various stages and each stage is important for the success of the treatment. Each stage is described briefly for the beginners.

ACCESS CAVITY PREPARATION

Access cavity preparation implies the creation of a space from occlusal table to canal orifice (s) so as to facilitate instrumentation, irrigation and obturation of the root canals. This is so significant in root canal therapy that it is described as gateway to success. The aim of the operator is to negotiate, prepare and obturate the canals. The proper access cavity, following basic principles of tooth preparation, without damaging the remaining tooth structure is important for achieving success in root canal therapy.

Objectives of Access Cavity Preparation

- To gain direct access to the apical foramen (not merely to the canal orifices).
- To facilitate removal of pulp tissue from coronal as well as radicular spaces.
- To facilitate instrumentation of the canal spaces, subsequently preparing and obturating the canals.
- To maintain structural integrity of the tooth as far as possible.

Points to Remember

- The initial entry should be made through occlusal or lingual surface and never through proximal surface.
- If we try to approach the pulp chamber and the canals through the proximal surface, the instruments that may be flexible, can bend at severe angles leading to ledge formation and even breakage of the instruments. Even otherwise, by doing so, the pulp tissue in the coronal aspect remains untouched, which leads to failure (Fig. 12.1).
- The rubber dam should be placed after initial access preparation so that the

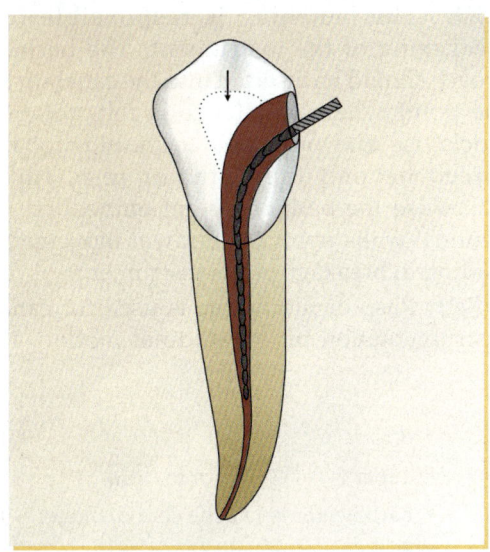

Fig. 12.1: *Wrong way to access preparation. Arrow shows untouched pulp tissue*

cementoenamel junction area of the concerned tooth and the adjacent teeth are visible.

- During 'reading' of radiograph, if the radio-lucency abruptly vanishes or diminishes in size, a bifurcation of the canal is suspected. Another radiograph at an angle of 20°–30° mesial/distal can help confirming the bifurcation.
- The radiograph should also be evaluated for overall configuration of the pulp chamber and the pulp horn, if any.
- The inclination of the roots in the jaws must be evaluated before access cavity preparation.

Before proceeding to access cavity preparation in different teeth, the basic knowledge of the root canal instruments used is mandatory. The routinely used instruments are:

Broach: Broach can be smooth or barbed. Earlier smooth broach was used as the first instrument to negotiate the canal; however, its place has been taken over by path finders.

Barbed broach is used for taking out the intracanal contents, whether vital pulp, cotton dressings or paper points (Fig. 12.2). It is a tapered instrument made from a stainless steel wire by notching it, producing barbs. Depending upon the configuration of barbs, the broaches can be designated as 'X', 'XX' and 'XXX'. This notching is responsible for weakening of the instrument. The barbed broach should be inserted into the canal up to the point where resistance is felt, rotated clockwise and outward. It should not be forced beyond the point of resistance; otherwise the barbs may get embedded in dentinal walls upon withdrawal movement, leading to breakage of the instrument.

Rasp: Rasp or rat tail file is used for canal instrumentation in longitudinal motion. Its

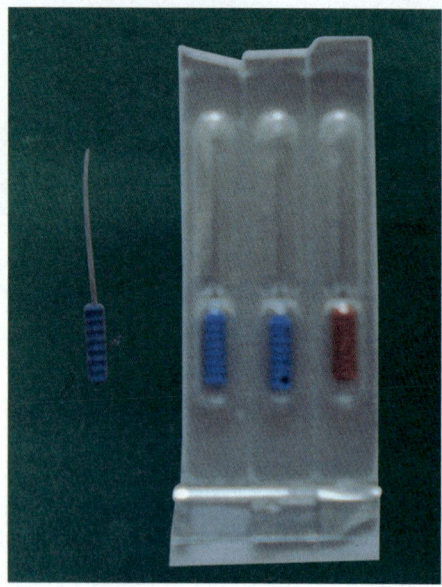

Fig. 12.2: *Barbed broaches*

barbs usually fall off in canal during instrumentation, so not preferred these days. Recently, two new instruments with cutting surface like that of rasps has been introduced, namely Rispi files and Sonic shaper. They have circumferential grooves rather than barbs coupled with smooth ends to avoid ledging.

Length of working portion is 10.0 mm in broach and rasp as compared to 16.0 mm in files and reamers.

Reamers: Reamers are used to prepare the root canals (Fig. 12.3). These are manufactured from a wire that is triangular in cross-section. The wire is held firmly at one end and the other end is twisted to form a spiral instrument. The triangular blank has an angle of 60° at each end, so sharp knife like edge is produced. The resultant instrument is sharp and flexible but susceptible to fracture. The cutting edge angle of reamer is 20°, so used with

Broach	Rasp
• Taper is 0.007– 0.01 mm/mm.	• Taper is 0.015– 0.02 mm/mm.
• Barb height is 1/2 the core diameter.	• Barb height is 1/3 the core diameter.
• Barbs are deep and sharp.	• Barbs are shallow and round.
• Weaker as compared to rasp.	• Stronger than broach.

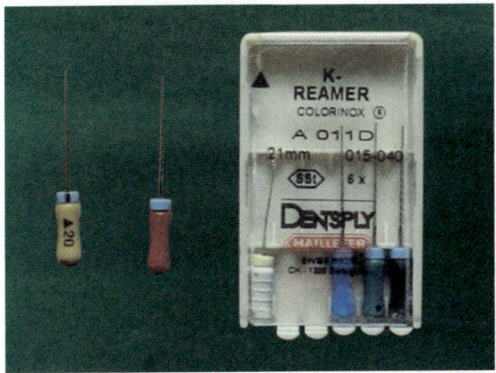

Fig. 12.3: *Reamers*

reaming motion, i.e. insert the instrument in the canal unit it binds; rotate it in clockwise direction giving one full rotation and then withdrawn. Such type of rotation will shave the dentin. Anticlockwise rotation, however, is used to insert any medicament in the canal.

Files: Different types of files are available (Fig. 12.4).

K-files: Most commonly used instrument for canal preparation. It is made from square blank of wire. The prefix 'K' is derived from 'Kerr' manufacturing company. It has more flutes per mm as compared to reamer, which makes it more cutting efficient. The files are less flexible. The cutting edge angle is 40°, so instrument can be used with reaming or filing motion. Reaming action includes inserting the file up to the point where it binds, give half a rotation, and withdraw. If the file is screwed in canal, chances of fracture increases.

K-flex files: These files are made from the wire which is diamond-shaped in cross-section. These are manufactured in order to overcome the drawbacks of K-files which include decreased flexibility which limit the use of K-files in curved canals. In diamond blank, two acute angles serve as cutting edges and two obtuse angles provide increased space for clearance of debris.

H-files (Hedstrom files): In H-file, the flutes resemble as if successively smaller triangles are placed one upon another. File is formed by grinding a single continuous round wire. Cutter gouges the wire in such a way that it produces triangular segments. As cutting edge angle is 60°, the instrument is used in withdrawal motion only. The instrument is relatively sharp and extremely efficient. H-files are indicated for wider canals and for removal of intracanal filling material like gutta-percha, etc. The drawbacks of these files are that the instrument is weak and liable to fracture.

The stainless steel files, though good in cutting lacks flexibility.

Ni-Ti files were introduced to make the files flexible. With the use of Ni-Ti files chances of strip perforation and apical transportation decrease.

Spreaders and Pluggers

These are the hand instruments used during obturation of root canals.

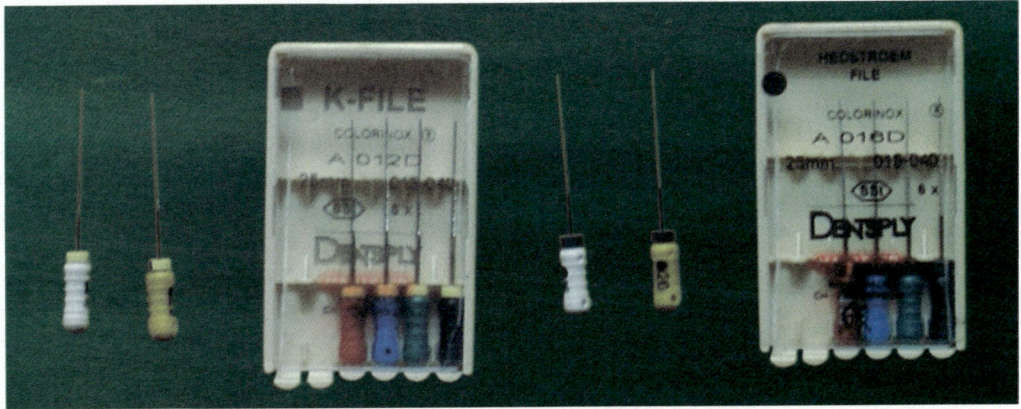

Fig. 12.4: *K-files and H-files*

Reamers	Files
• Made from triangular blank of wire.	• Made from square blank of wire.
• No. of flutes are 1–1½ per mm.	• No. of flutes are 1½ – 2½ per mm.
• Rake angle is 60° (sharp).	• Rake angle is 90° (less sharp).
• Used with reaming motion.	• Can be used with reaming or rasping motion.
• Chip space is 60%.	• Chip space is 36% so does not allow much removal of loosened material.
• Reaming action produces canals that are relatively round in shape.	• Filing action produces canals that are relatively irregular in shape.
• Less efficient.	• More efficient.
• More flexible.	• Less flexible.
• Failure rate is higher.	• Failure rate is less.

Root canal spreaders are tapered, pointed metal instruments with a smooth surface. They are used for lateral condensation of filling material in the root canal. These are available in different sizes with different taper. They can have a long or short handles. Spreaders with short handle are called finger spreaders (Fig. 12.5).

Root canal pluggers are slightly tapered and flat ended metal instruments with smooth surface, used for vertical condensation of filling material (Fig. 12.6). Like that of spreaders, these can have short or long

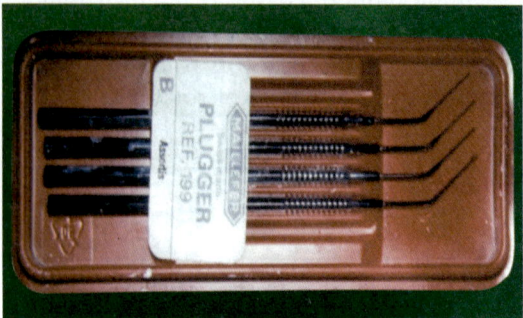

Fig. 12.6: *Hand pluggers*

handles. One with short handle is called finger plugger.

ACCESS CAVITY PREPARATION FOR MAXILLARY TEETH

Maxillary Anteriors

• In labiolingual section, the pulp cavity comes to a point near the incisal edge, becomes wider at the centre and then tapers at the cervical area, which continues up to apex.

• In mesiodistal section, the pulp cavity is wider in the centre, with pulp horns extending towards the incisal area. The canal tapers from center to cervical area and up to apex. The configuration of pulp cavity both labiolingually and mesiodistally is almost same in maxillary lateral incisors and canines.

Steps of access cavity preparation (applicable for all anterior teeth) (Fig. 12.7)

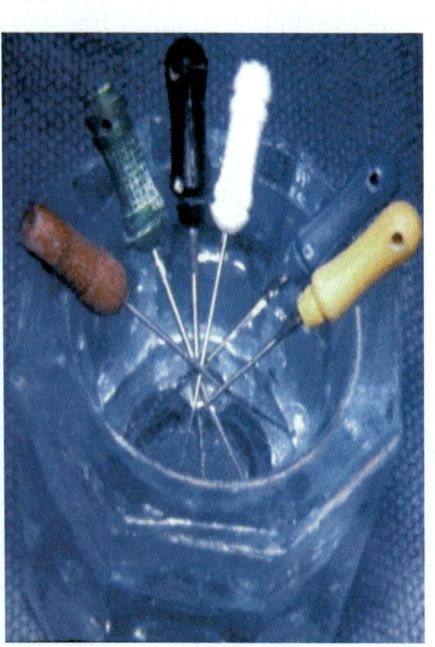

Fig. 12.5: *Finger spreaders*

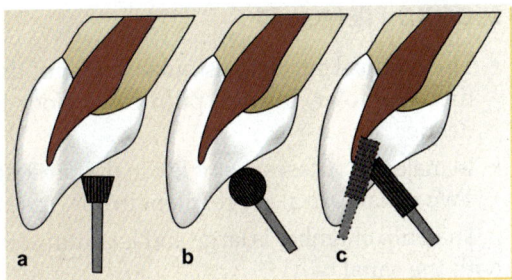

Fig. 12.7a to c: *Steps for maxillary anterior teeth. (a) Inverted cone bur for nick, (b) round bur to reach dentin, (c) fissure bur to open pulp chamber and for widening of preparation*

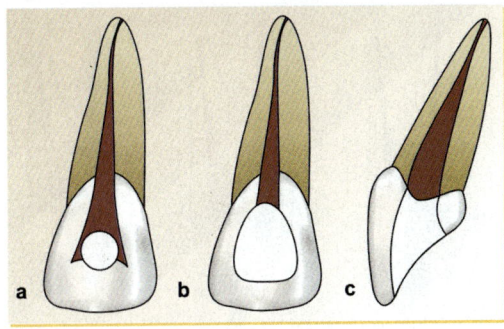

Fig. 12.8a to c: *Access preparation. (a) Wrong (pulp tissue left), (b) and (c) right (no pulp tissue)*

- The first step is to give a "nick" just below the cingulum in the centre of the lingual surface with the help of an inverted cone bur, keeping the bur perpendicular to the surface. The nick prevents slipping of the bur into the gingival sulcus.

- Through this 'nick', penetrate into dentin with the help of appropriate round bur.

- Once dentin is reached, the bur is held parallel to the long axis of the tooth until the pulp chamber is reached.

- The maxillary central incisor is proclined 5–10° in the jaw. Therefore, the bur should be angled accordingly, to be parallel to the long axis of the tooth. This angle is known as 'access angle'.

- The palatal inclination of lateral incisor is 25° and that of canines is 17°. Usually these teeth are distally tilted. Care should be taken during access cavity preparation of these teeth.

- The access is enlarged both labiolingually and mesiodistally.

  Pulp tissue remnants should not be left in the pulp chamber, which may discolour the remaining tooth structure and subsequently failure of the root canal therapy (Fig. 12.8).

  In the labiolingual direction, labial and lingual triangles need to be removed.

  In the mesiodistal direction, pulp horns should be uncovered.

- The extensions of pulp horns under each mesial and distal angle should be checked.

- It is important to note that in all incisors, a better straight line access can be achieved through an incisal access cavity; the lingual approach is used in order to maintain as much tooth structure on labial surface as possible for esthetic reasons.

- But in the cases where tooth has to be restored with crown, the endodontic access is made through labial or incisal surface as required.

FIRST PREMOLAR

- In the labiolingual section, pulp horn usually extend farther incisally under the buccal cusp as latter is usually better developed than the lingual cusp.

- In mesiodistal section, pulp horns appear blunt and pulp chamber is in continuation with the root canals.

- Mostly two canals are present (more than 60%) and the possibility of third canal is also not uncommon.

Steps of Access Cavity Preparation

- The access cavity is prepared using round bur starting from centre of the fossa and moving to buccal and palatal sides. The oval shape is achieved.

- An appropriate round bur is used to open into the pulp chamber. The tactile sense will feel 'dropping the bur' when the pulp chamber is reached. In chronic cases and also where the pulp is calcified, such a 'drop' is not felt. The tapered fissure bur is then used to penetrate deep and completely

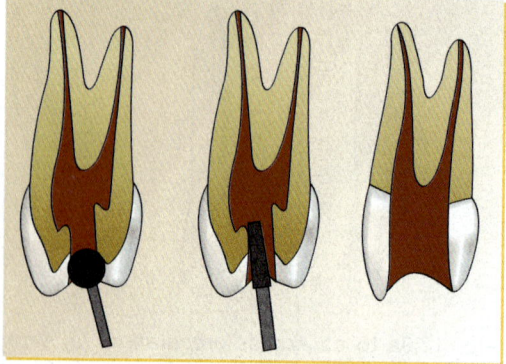

Fig. 12.9: *Stages of opening of posterior teeth*

deroof the chamber. Care must be exercised not to injure the furcation area (Fig. 12.9).

- After penetrating the pulp chamber the orifices can be located using fine instruments.
- The buccal canal lies beneath the buccal cusp and the palatal canal lies beneath the palatal cusp.
- The lumen of the palatal canal is larger than that of buccal canal. The buccal canal is generally more difficult to negotiate.
- One should explore the possibility of third canal, which is usually in mesiobuccal direction.
- The shape of the access cavity is depicted in Fig. 12.10

SECOND PREMOLAR

- The occlusal surface is similar to that of the first premolar, but the pulp canal floor is deeper.
- In majority of cases, a single canal is present. Two canals are also prevalent in 30% cases.

The pulp chamber is large and is continuous with the canal.

At the cervical level, the pulp cavity is elliptical and wide buccolingually.

Steps of Access Cavity Preparation

- The access cavity preparation is same as for maxillary first premolar.
- Usually one canal is present in the centre; however, if one canal is found and not in centre, there is possibility of second root canal.
- The two canals, if present, are palatal and buccal.
- Very rarely third canal can also be present.
- The shape of the access cavity is depicted in Fig. 12.11.

FIRST MOLAR

- The maxillary first molar has three separate roots—two buccal and one palatal with one canal in each root. Any root can have extra

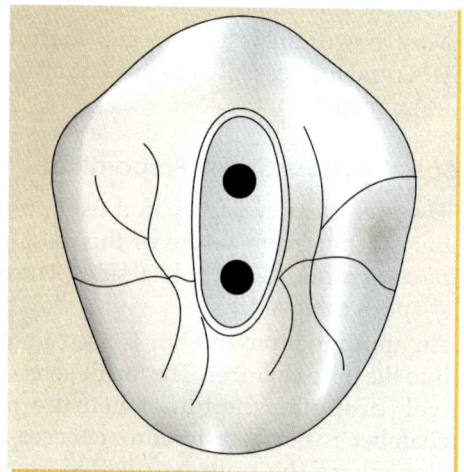

Fig. 12.10: *Shape of access cavity preparation for maxillary first premolar*

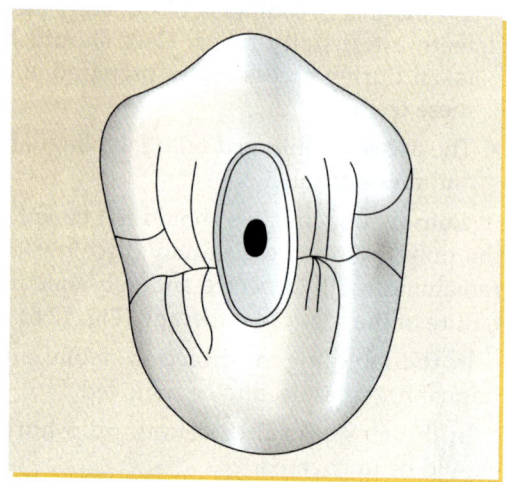

Fig. 12.11: *Shape of access cavity preparation for maxillary second premolar*

canal, with more chances in mesiobuccal root.

- The pulp chamber is in mesial half of the tooth.
- The palatal canal is wider than either of the buccal canals.

Steps of Access Cavity Preparation

- Access cavity preparation should be initiated in the mesial fossa.
- The tapered fissure bur is used and extended towards the mesiopalatal cusp as the orifice of palatal canal is present beneath the mesiopalatal cusp.
- The orifice of mesiobuccal canal is also located beneath the mesiobuccal cusp but the distobuccal canal orifice does not relate to its cusp. It is usually located by means of its relation to the mesiobuccal orifice and is found approximately 2.0 to 3.0 mm to the distal and slightly to the palatal aspect of the mesiobuccal orifice.
- With the help of fine instruments, the orifice of palatal canal is located, followed by other two canals.
- The access cavity is given a quadrilateral shape.
- The mesiobuccal root shows a second canal called MB2 which is found 1.0–2.0 mm palatal to the main mesiobuccal canal.
- Very rarely the palatal and the distobuccal roots can have extra root canals.
- The access cavity is kept mesial to the oblique ridge. There is no need to sacrifice the oblique ridge in preparing the access cavity as all orifices of canals lie in the mesial three-fifths of the crown.
- The shape of the access cavity is depicted in Fig. 12.12

SECOND MOLAR

- Maxillary second molar varies in shape. It can be three rooted, two rooted and even single rooted. Subsequently, the canals can be three as in first molar and two or one depending upon the number of roots.
- Extra canals can also be present in any root, as are prevalent in mesiobuccal root.

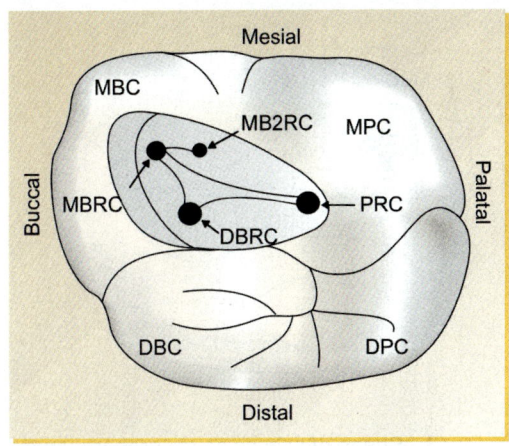

Fig. 12.12: *Shape of access cavity preparation for maxillary first molar. MBRC: mesiobuccal root canal; DBRC: distobuccal root canal; MB2RC: mesiobuccal 2 root canal; PRC: palatal root canal*

Steps of Access Cavity Preparation

- The radiograph should thoroughly be evaluated before starting the access cavity preparation. Semi-parallel technique can be followed if malar prominence interferes in the proper viewing of the root canals.
- The access cavity is prepared in the same manner and shape as for the first molar. The access is from the mesial side only.
- The mesiobuccal canal and root are not as long buccolingually as those of the first molar.
- The mesiobuccal canal if present, pose difficulties in negotiation, because of distally placed tooth.
- The shape of the access cavity is depicted in Fig. 12.13.

ACCESS CAVITY PREPARATION FOR MANDIBULAR TEETH

Mandibular Anteriors

The root canal is usually small and rounded mesiodistally and slightly flat in labiolingual direction. The mandibular incisors may have second root canal (40% incidence). The incisors and canines are lingually tilted. The lateral incisors and canines are also distally tilted.

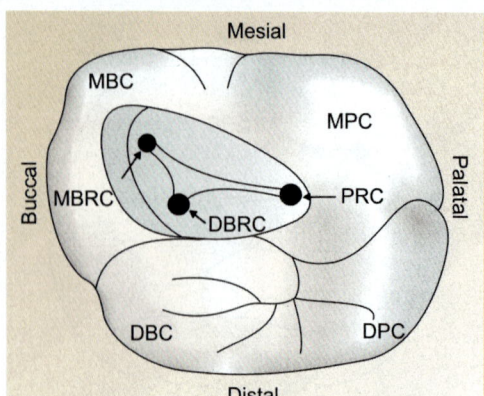

Fig. 12.13: *Shape of access cavity preparation for maxillary second molar. MBRC: mesiobuccal root canal; DBRC: distobuccal root canal; PRC: palatal root canal*

Steps of Access Cavity Preparation (Fig. 12.14)

- Just above the cingulum a small 'nick' is given with the inverted cone bur perpendicular to the surface. Only enamel is penetrated at this time (as in maxillary incisors).
- Through the nick, the access cavity is deepened using round bur.
- Same bur can be used or with fissure bur, the cavity is extended mesiodistally to include the pulp chamber.
- Final access cavity shape is ovoid, funnel shaped which is wider labiolingually.

- The preparation is similar for lateral incisors and canines.
- The bifurcated canals are more prevalent in canines.

MANDIBULAR FIRST PREMOLAR

- The mandibular first premolar resembles canine; the cingulum simulates the lingual cusp.
- The mesiolingual developmental groove makes the tooth asymmetrical.
- The crown is lingually tilted by 45°. The distal inclination is approximately 10°. The bifurcated root canals are quite prevalent in first premolar.

Steps of Access Cavity Preparation

- The preparation is started in the middle of the central groove using round/fissure bur.
- The bur is extended more buccally and less lingually.
  The occlusal opening is widened buccolingually to twice the width of the bur to allow room for exploration.
- The canal is located with the help of an explorer. Working from inside to outside, the roof of the pulp chamber is completely removed with appropriate burs.
- Final preparation is ovoid and tapered from the occlusal downwards providing a straight line access to the canal (Fig. 12.15).

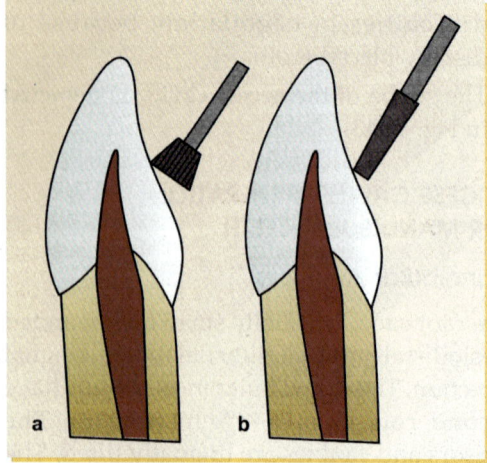

Fig. 12.14a and b: *Steps for mandibular anterior teeth*

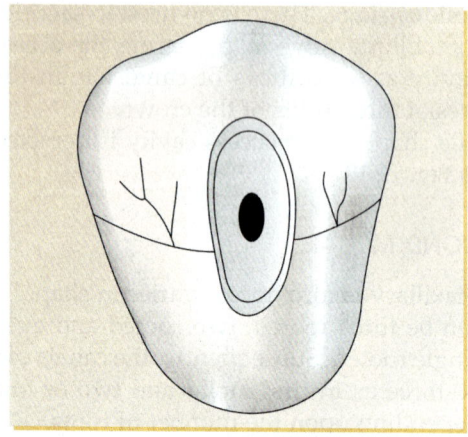

Fig. 12.15: *Shape of access cavity preparation for mandibular first premolar*

MANDIBULAR SECOND PREMOLAR

- The mandibular second premolar can be of three cusp type or two cusp type.
- The crown is distally and lingually inclined, though not as much as first premolar. Lingual pulp horn is quite prominent.

Steps of Access Cavity Preparation

- Access cavity is prepared in the same manner as for first premolar.
- It usually has one root and one well-centered canal; but may have bifurcated canals.
- Access is made ovoid, wider in the bucco-lingual dimensions (Fig. 12.16).

MANDIBULAR FIRST MOLAR

- Mandibular first molar generally has two distinct roots, one mesial and the other distal. Three canals are usually present—one in distal root and two in mesial root, i.e. mesiobuccal and mesiolingual.
- The buccolingual section reveals that the pulp chamber is in the centre of the crown and that the distal canal is ribbon shaped, whereas the mesial canals are thin.

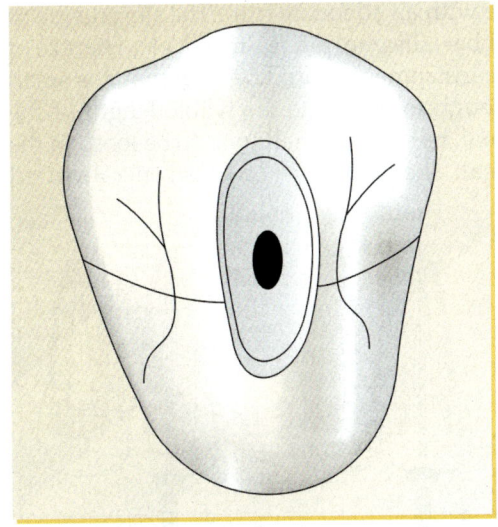

Fig. 12.16: *Shape of access cavity preparation for mandibular second premolar*

Steps of Access Cavity Preparation

- General outline of the access cavity is trapezoidal. The buccal and lingual sides are of approximately the same configuration and taper towards each other distally.
- The access cavity preparation is started just mesial to the central pit. Since the tooth is lingually and mesially inclined, the bur should mimic these angulations. The access cavity is confined to mesial half of the crown.
- The orifice of the distal canal lies beneath the central pit. It is generally large and slightly elliptical.
- The mesiolingual canal lies beneath the mesial pit. The mesiobuccal canal lies beneath the mesiobuccal cusp. The orifices are often connected by a groove which helps to locate both canals.
- An appropriate bur is used to remove the roof of the pulp chamber guiding the bur from inside to outside.
- It should be kept in mind that a wider access cavity to locate extra canals is better than ignoring these for the sake of a 'conservative' preparation, which may lead to failure.
- The shape of the access cavity is depicted in Fig. 12.17.

MANDIBULAR SECOND MOLAR

- The second molar is inclined more lingually than the first molar; therefore the access preparation should correspond to the tilt of the tooth.

Steps of Access Cavity Preparation

- Access cavity is prepared in the same way as in the case of a first molar.
- There may be three root canals as in first molar or in majority only two canals are present.
- C-shape canal configuration is quite common in mandibular second molar.
- The shape of the access cavity is depicted in Fig. 12.18.

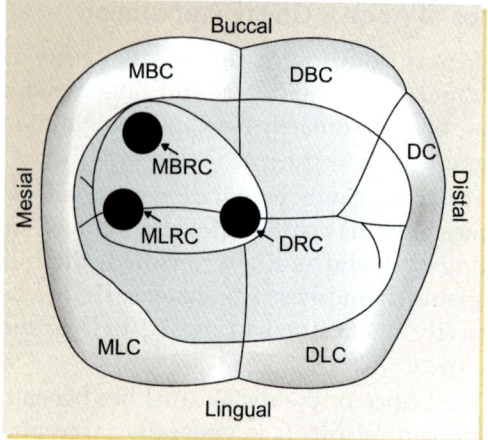

Fig. 12.17: *Shape of access cavity preparation for mandibular first molar. MBRC: mesiobuccal root canal; MLRC: mesiolingual root canal; DRC: distal root canal*

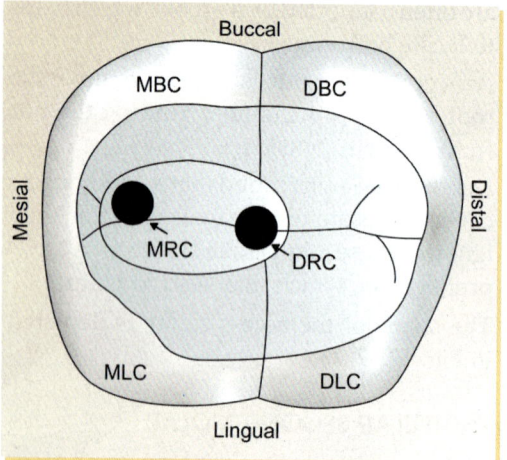

Fig. 12.18: *Shape of access cavity preparation for mandibular second molar. MRC: mesial root canal; DRC: distal root canal*

WORKING LENGTH MEASUREMENT

The working length implies the area beyond which the instrumentation is not to be carried out. The instruments and the obturating materials are confined up to the apical constriction of the root canal or the dentino-cementum junction. The length of the root canal from the reference point up to the apical constriction is the working length.

There are various materials, techniques and gadgets available for measuring the working length. The most acceptable and the routinely followed method is the Ingle's method, which is described for the beginners (Fig. 12.19).

Ingle's Method

Ingle's method is the modified radiographic method. A good undistorted preoperative radiograph is required for reference. The plane of reference in the concerned tooth should be definite and reproducible. Any plane of reference like unsupported tooth structure that can be lost should not be included but reduced to sound tooth structure. The incisal edges of the anterior teeth and cusp tips of the posterior teeth is definitive and repeatable plane of reference.

The instrument that is required to determine the working length is generally a stainless steel file with an adequate stop. The stop can be of rubber, silicone, plastic, metal, etc. The size of the instrument should be such that it is small enough to negotiate the whole length of the canal, but not so small so as to be loose in the canal. The file size 15 or 20 is generally used

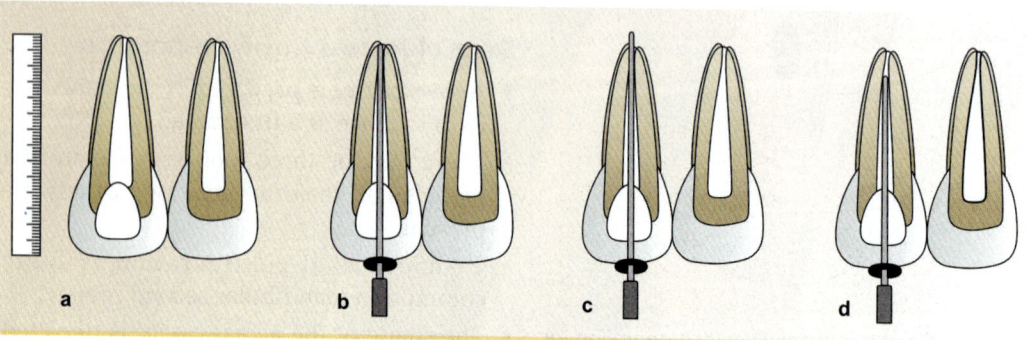

Fig. 12.19a to d: *Ingle's method*

since these can wiggle through the pulpal tissue until reach the apex.

Procedure

1. Measure the tooth length on the pre-operative radiograph.
2. Select an instrument with stop at that length.
3. Place the instrument in the canal until the stop is at the plane of reference point.
4. Get another radiograph with the selected instrument inside the canal.
5. Three possibilities can be evident. One, the tip of the instrument is up to the apical end of the root. Second, the instrument goes beyond the apical end and third, the instrument is falling short of the apical end. In case of first possibility the length remains the same; in case of second possibility, the length of the instrument extending beyond the apical end is to be subtracted from the premeasured length. In case of third possibility the length of the instrument falling short is to be added to that length.

The length so achieved is the length of the root. Another 1.0–1.5 mm is to be subtracted to achieve the working length.

In curved canals, as preparation proceeds, the curved canals straighten out and approximately 1.0 mm of the length may be lost further. Therefore, the length should be reaffirmed in cases with curved canals.

When two canals may superimpose in one radiograph, two individual radiographs may be taken. Alternatively take another radiograph using slightly horizontal mesial/distal angulation. This exposes both the canals on the same radiograph.

For identification of the canal, Clarke's rule is followed, i.e. MBD; when X-rays are directed from the mesial, the buccal canal is more towards the distal and MLM; when X-rays are directed from the mesial, the lingual canal is more towards the mesial.

ROOT CANAL PREPARATION

The root canal preparation envisages cleaning the canal of all debris and shaping the same in such a manner so as to facilitate proper obturation. Earlier the term 'cleaning and shaping' was used. The necrosed pulp along with dentin which harbour the bacteria is to be cleaned. Thereafter the canal is given a shape conducive for receiving the gutta-percha or other obturation material. Various authors have described alternative techniques for preparation of root canals; only commonly used technique is described here for the beginners.

1. Step-Back Technique

The step-back technique is also known as serial root canal preparation. As the name indicates the preparation is carried out in steps, starting from apical end to coronal end (Fig. 12.20). The technique is divided into two phases:

a. Phase I is the apical preparation starting at the apical constriction.
b. Phase II is the preparation of the remaining canal, gradually stepping-back with increasing instrument sizes. The continuous taper is achieved from apex to cervical end.

Steps

- After the access cavity preparation, the canal(s) is explored using pathfinder or fine instrument.
- Working length is established preferably using Ingle's method.
- The first active instrument with 0.02% taper is inserted till the working length.
- The instrument that snuggly fits at apical constriction is called initial apical file (IAF).
- Starting with initial apical file, the files are used in 'watch winding' motion, two or three quarter turns clockwise-counter clockwise and then retracted. The canals are thoroughly irrigated. The procedure is repeated until the instrument is loose in position.
- Then the next size K-file is used with established working length.
- The process is continued till the apical constriction is prepared and free of all necrosed substrate responsible for bacterial growth.

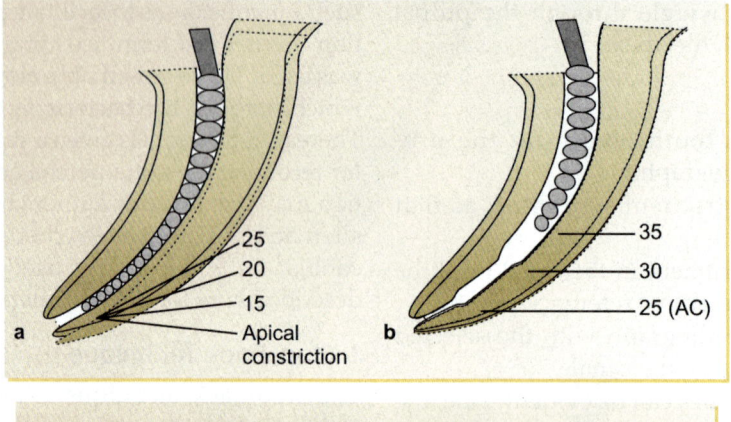

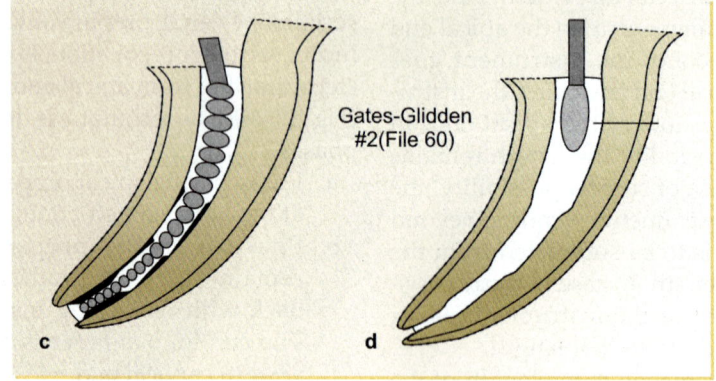

Fig. 12.20a to d: *Step back technique. (a) Enlarging apical constriction, (b) moving 1 mm coronally using large number of the instrument, (c) recapitulating the prepared canal, (d) enlarging coronal end with Gates-Glidden bur*

- After the apical preparation, next size file is used, 1.0 mm short of the actual working length.
- Next instrument is used 2.0 mm short of the working length.
- Recapitulation, i.e. sequential re-entry of each previous instrument to the actual working length is carried out to ensure the patency of the canal followed by irrigation.
- The process is continued stepping back 1.0 mm at each time with larger instruments.
- Coronal portions are prepared with Gates-Glidden drills/orifice opener.
- The canal is finally refined to achieve the desired taper from the apical constriction.

2. Crown-Down Technique

It is also known as Step-Down technique. Gates-Glidden drills and larger files are used first to prepare the coronal two-thirds of the canals and then progressively smaller files are used in coronal to apical direction (Fig. 12.21).

Advantages

- Allows effective irrigation and hence the danger of pushing the debris beyond the apex is reduced.
- Holds larger volume of irrigant and hence helps in dissolution of pulp tissue in the apical and lateral canals.
- Working length is less likely to change during apical instrumentation.
- Reduces the risk of instrument fracture.

Procedure

- The prepared access cavity is irrigated and the canal(s) patency is determined using fine instruments.
- An appropriate size file is inserted up to curvature and the length is measured. This

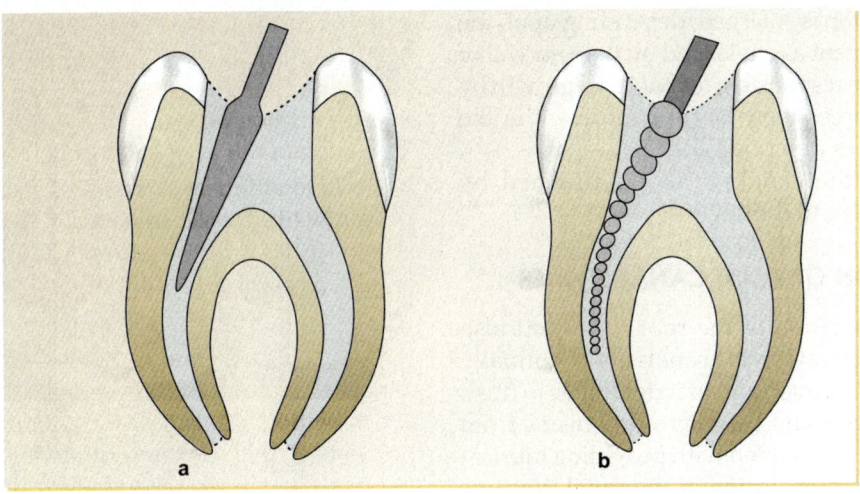

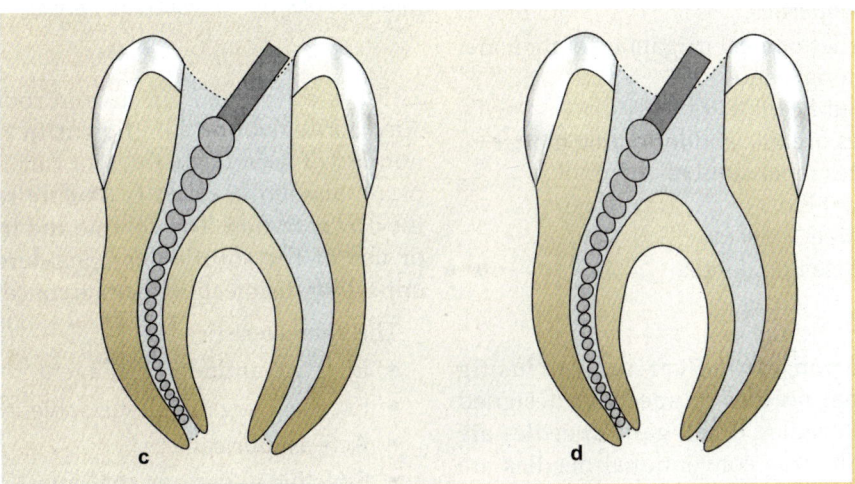

Fig. 12.21a to d: *Crown down technique. (a) Preparing coronal one third, (b) moving apically preparing middle half using small, (c) preparing apical area, (d) process repeated with larger number instrument, if required*

is known as radicular access length (RAL). Alternatively, the canal is divided into three parts. The coronal one-third is taken as radicular access length.

- Coronal portion is prepared using Gates-Glidden drills or corresponding files to radicular access length.
- Provisional working length is established from preoperative radiograph at a point 3.0 mm short of radiographic apex.
- The lesser number file is inserted and rotated clockwise slightly beyond radicular

access length until resistance is felt and the canal is prepared till the instrument is loose.

- The process is repeated till provisional working length is reached.
- Take a radiograph with the file at the provisional working length and estimate the true working length.
- Continue stepping down with smaller files to the true working length. The file that fits snuggly at the true working length is the initial apical file (IAF).

- Apical stop is enlarged, depending upon the requirement as envisaged by the removal of substrate responsible for bacterial growth by using successively larger instrument in the manner as described above.
- Finally the canal walls are finished by circumferential filing.

IRRIGATION OF ROOT CANAL SPACES

After preparation of the root canal and also during preparation, the canals are continually irrigated. The main aim of irrigation is to flush out the debris and the micro-organisms from the root canal, coupled with providing lubrication for the preparation of the canal. Various irrigating solutions are available, having different properties.

The properties of ideal irrigation solution are:
- Antibacterial action
- Acts as lubricant
- Dissolves organic and inorganic matter
- Stimulates repair process
- Biocompatible
- Substantive
- Can diffuse into dentin

Procedure

The irrigation can be carried out using conventional needles or specially designed perforated needles. Small gauze needles are preferred. In case conventional needles are used, the needle should be pushed half way through the root canal. Once the irrigating solution is pushed, it irrigates the apical half of the root canal (Fig. 12.22).

In case perforated needles are used, these can be pushed up to apical end. The irrigation is carried out all along the walls because of the perforation. The apical end of the needle is closed; therefore, no chance of the irrigating solution being pushed out of the apical foramen.

The commonly used irrigating solutions are:

1. Sodium Hypochlorite

Different concentration of sodium hypochlorite is being used as irrigating solution. 0.5–5.25% sodium hypochlorite can be used; however,

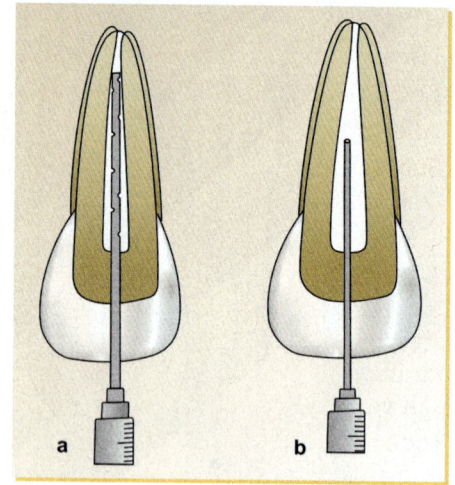

Fig. 12.22a and b: *Irrigating technique. (a) Perforated needle, (b) conventional needle*

2.25% is considered effective in routine use. Any concentration is efficient in reducing number of bacteria in the root canal, but the tissue dissolving effect is directly related to the concentration. The volume and frequency of use of the solution is considered more critical for disinfection than its concentration.

The characteristics are:
- Effective antimicrobial agent
- Excellent organic tissue solvent
- Acts as lubricant
- Effective in various concentration

Limitations
- Not effective against E. *faecalis*
- Not substantive
- Ineffective in smear layer removal
- Toxic to soft tissues
- Unpleasant odour

2. Chlorhexidine

0.1–0.2% chlorhexidine is used in routine as an irrigating solution. The cationic properties of chlorhexidine allow the solution to bind electrostatically to the root surface, which can be released slowly in the environment. This property of 'substantivity' makes chlorhexidine useful irrigating solution.

The properties are:
- Useful in low concentration
- Low level of tissue toxicity
- Allergic reaction are rare
- Substantivity

3. EDTA

Ethylenediamine tetra-acetic acid (concentration: 17%) is a chelating agent used to dissolve the inorganic content of infected dentin. It can be used to effectively navigate through very fine and calcified canals.

A wide range of irrigants are available with effective antibacterial, lubricating and tissue dissolving properties. Few of them are:
- MTAD
- Q Mix
- Nano-irrigants

ROOT CANAL OBTURATION

After the root canal is prepared, irrigated and dried, the space so achieved is obturated by solid or semisolid materials. Various materials and different techniques are utilized to obturate the canal spaces; however, for the beginners, only lateral compaction method utilizing gutta-percha is described. This is the most common technique and material, which is followed in routine by dental professionals.

Why to Obturate

- Prevents percolation and microleakage of periapical exudate into root canal space.
- Prevents reinfection of root canal during transient bacteraemia.
- Creates favourable environment for the process of healing.

When to Obturate

- Tooth is asymptomatic, i.e. no pain or tenderness.
- Canal is dry, i.e. no excessive exudates or seepage
- Sinus tract, if present has healed.
- Coronal seal is intact.

Requirements of an Ideal Obturating Material

- Dimensionally stable.
- Able to seal the canal in three dimensions.
- Should not irritate periapical tissues.
- Bactericidal.
- Radio-opaque.
- Unaffected by tissue fluid.
- Easily removed, if required.

Lateral Compaction Technique

Lateral compaction/condensation technique is the most commonly used technique. In this technique, root canal is coated with sealer, followed by placement of a gutta-percha point that is laterally compacted by spreader to make space for accessory points. The final mass is severed at the canal orifice with a hot instrument and the gutta-percha is compacted vertically at the coronal orifice.

The procedure is carried out following the steps as under:

1. Drying the root canal

The canal should be thoroughly dried using paper points before obturation.

2. Selection of master gutta-percha

As the gutta-percha is available in standardized sizes, the selected size should match the size of the last instrument used at the apical constriction (Figs 12.23 to 12.26).

- The selected gutta-percha point is measured and marked to the actual working length. The master cone is tried in the wet canal and should coincide with the reference point on the tooth. If the point goes beyond the working length, the next (bigger) size gutta-percha point should be used. If that point does not reach the working length, then the tip of the previous gutta-percha should be cut off and tried again.
- The gutta-percha point at this junction should not be loose and resist the removal. This resistance to removal of the gutta-percha is known as TUGBACK.
- Finally the length and extent of gutta-percha point can be confirmed with radiographs.

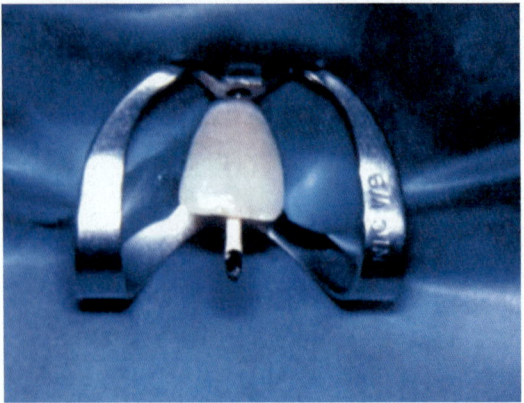

Fig. 12.23: *Selecting master gutta-percha point*

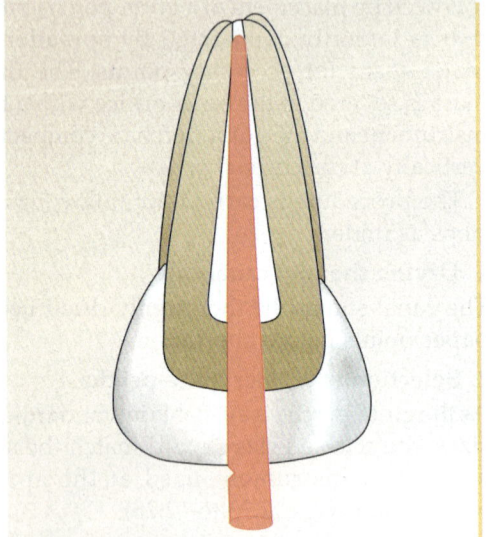

Fig. 12.24: *Selecting master gutta-percha point (diagrammatic)*

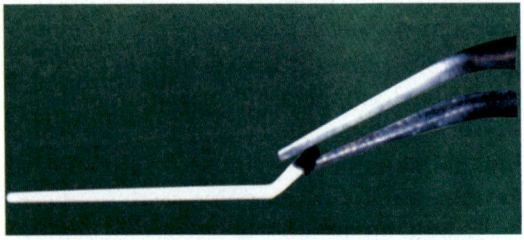

Fig. 12.25: *Giving nick to the gutta-percha*

3. Mixing and placement of the sealer

Various sealers are available; the commonly used are:

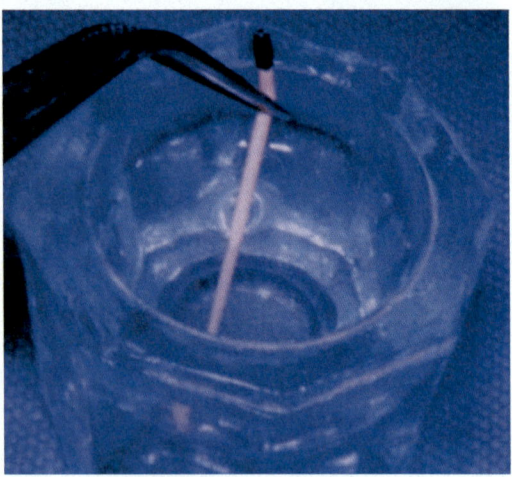

Fig. 12.26: *Dipping gutta-percha in alcohol or sodium hypochlorite solution*

- Zinc oxide eugenol
- Non-eugenol zinc oxide
- Calcium hydroxide
- Resins
- Iodoform paste

The sealers help to fill the minor irregularities in the canal walls and accessory canals, if present. They also act as lubricants and binding agents.

The sealer should be mixed on a sterile glass slab to a creamy consistency. It should string out at least an inch when the spatula is lifted from the mix or it should be held for 10 seconds on an inverted spatula without dropping off.

Sealer can be placed in the canal using the master gutta-percha cone, rotating the same clockwise in the canal; alternatively the sealer can be placed using file or reamer in anticlockwise direction (Figs 12.27 and 12.28).

4. Selection and use of spreaders

Spreaders are available in different sizes and tapers. The spreaders' size should be such that it is loose within the canal and should not penetrate beyond the apex. The force applied by the spreader should be against the gutta-percha. The initial spreader should be 2.0–3.0 mm short of working length. The spreaders

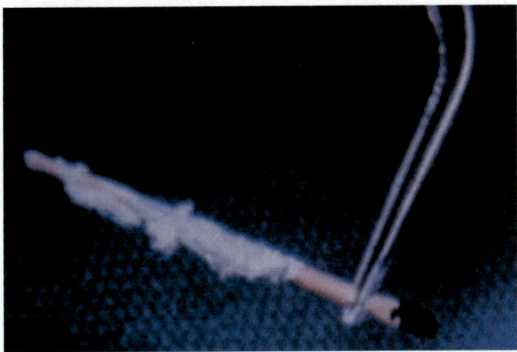

Fig. 12.27: *Sealer entrapment with master gutta-percha*

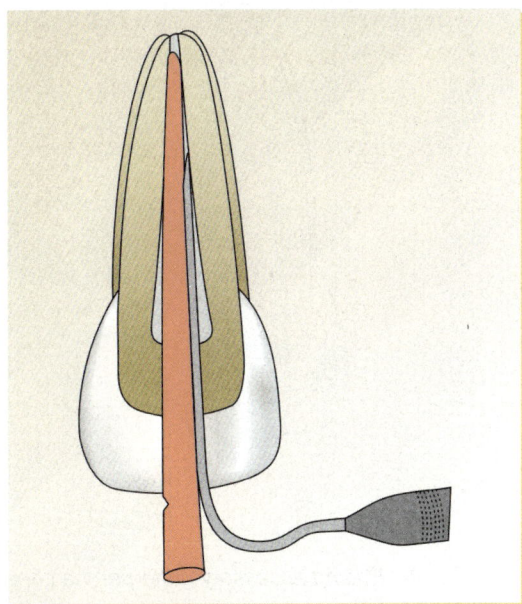

Fig. 12.29: *Putting spreader along the master gutta-percha (diagrammatic)*

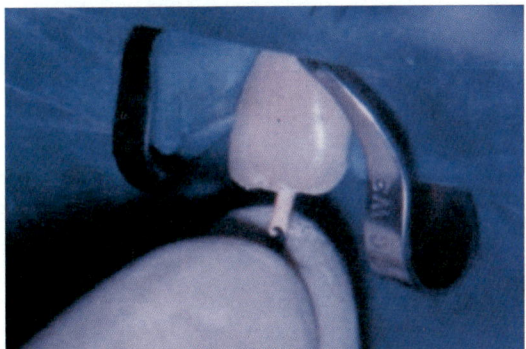

Fig. 12.28: *Applying sealer in the root canal*

should be kept in the root canal for 20 seconds so that the requisite compaction is achieved, prior to pushing accessory gutta-percha cones. The process is repeated till the canal is hermetically compacted (Figs 12.29 to 12.33).

5. Finally the gutta-percha points hanging out of the coronal end are seared off using hot burnishers. The remaining gutta-percha is condensed in the canal orifices (Figs 12.34 to 12.36).

6. The access cavity is filled with suitable restorative material.

7. Radiograph is taken to confirm the obturation (Figs 12.37 to 12.39).

Procedural Errors

Indifferent knowledge of internal anatomy of tooth often leads to procedural errors which become task for the clinician to manage.

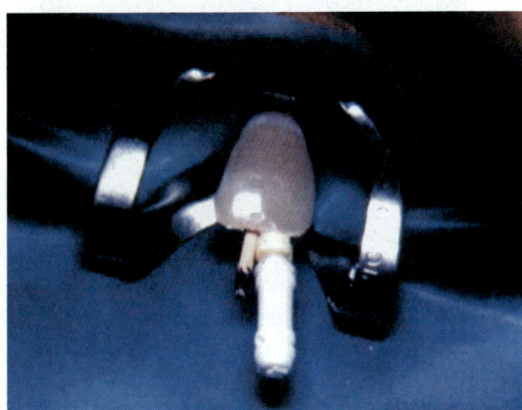

Fig. 12.30: *Putting spreader along the master gutta-percha*

Various procedural errors are:
1. Canal blockage
2. Canal transportation
3. Ledge formation
4. Perforation

1. Canal Blockage

A canal may get blocked by the dentinal debris or temporary filling material, if not irrigated

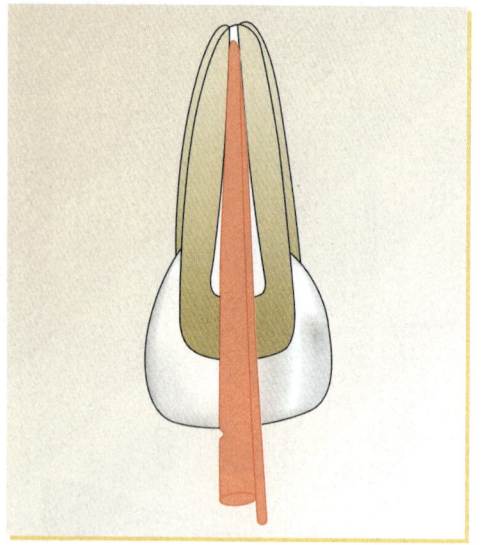

Fig. 12.31: *Putting accessory gutta-percha cones (diagrammatic)*

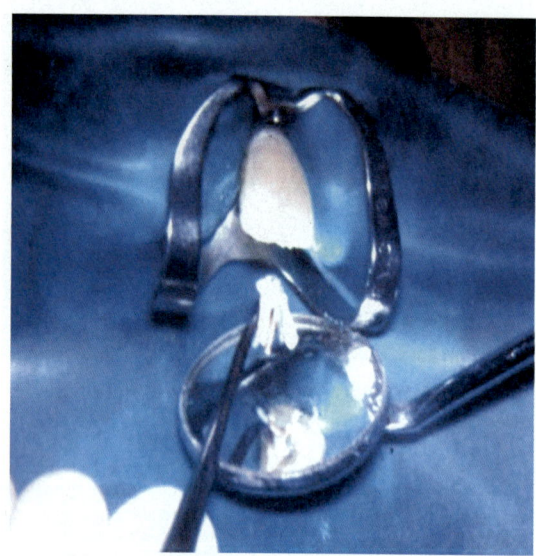

Fig. 12.34: *Removing extra gutta-percha*

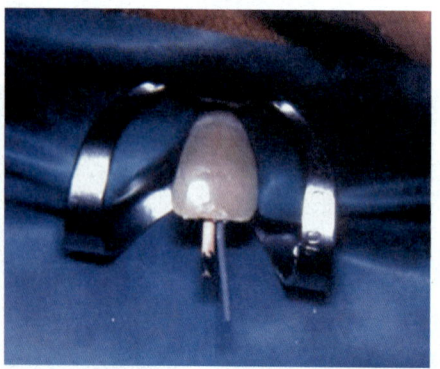

Fig. 12.32: *Putting accessory gutta-percha cones*

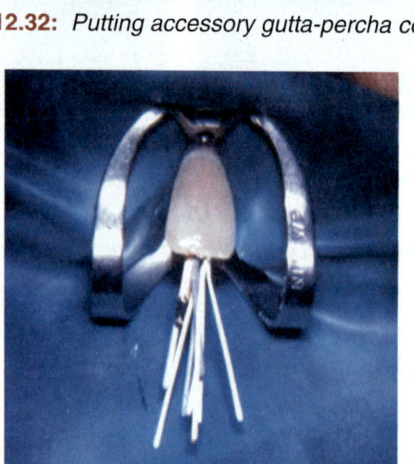

Fig. 12.33: *Filling remaining canal space with accessory cones*

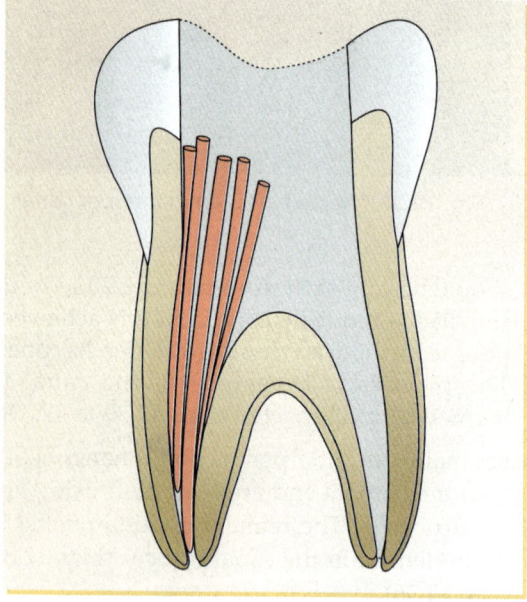

Fig. 12.35: *Removing hanging gutta-percha (diagrammatic)*

properly leading to shortening of working length (Fig. 12.40).

2. Canal Transportation

It is mandatory to maintain the shape of canal during root canal preparation. The apical

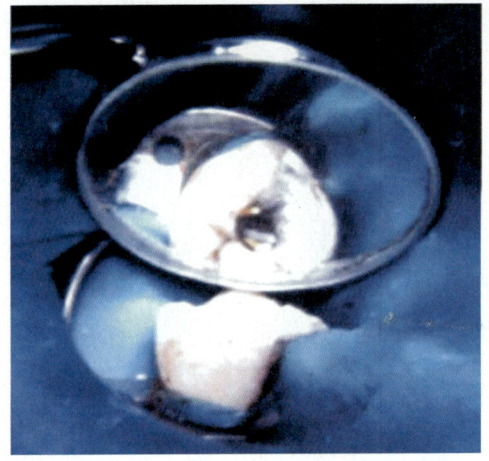

Fig. 12.36: *Removing hanging gutta-percha*

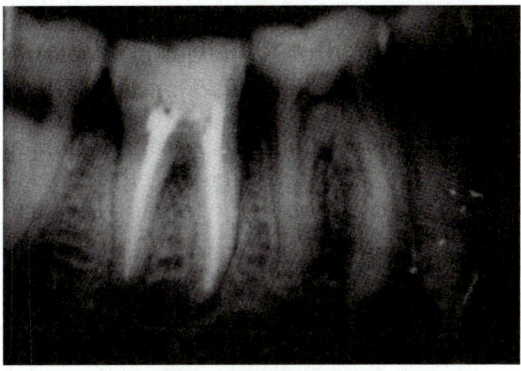

Fig. 12.39: *Completed obturation*

terminus may get deviated due to improper instrumentation.

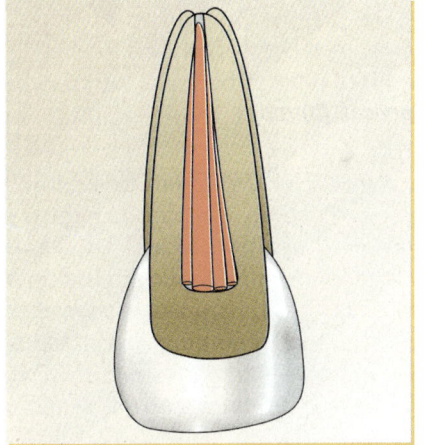

Fig. 12.37: *Completed obturation (diagrammatic)*

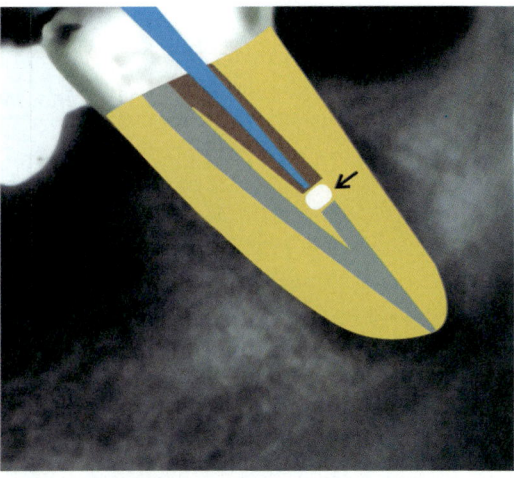

Fig. 12.40: *Canal blockage*

3. Ledge Formation

When the canal is gouged resulted in short canal instrumentation in otherwise patent canal, it is known as ledging. It is usually created at the beginning of curvature when root canal instrument is used without pre-curving or using excessive amount of apical pressure.

4. Perforation

Perforation is the iatrogenic communication of root space with periodontal tissues. It can occur during the preparation of an access cavity or cleaning and shaping of the root canal system (Fig. 12.41a and b).

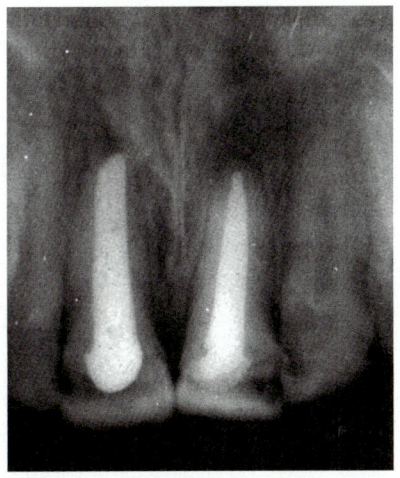

Fig. 12.38: *Completed obturation*

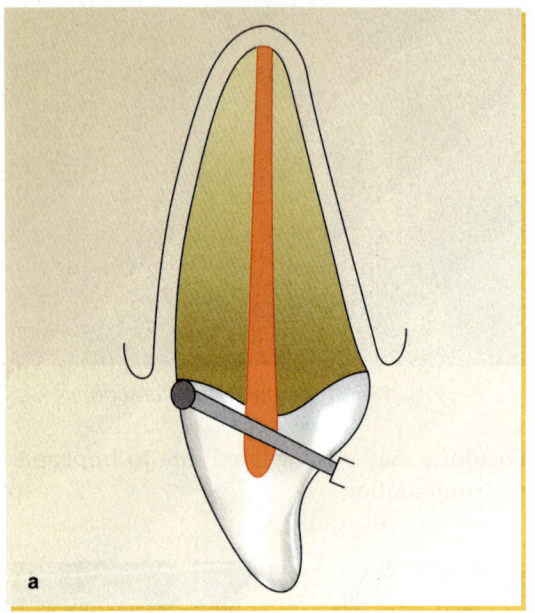 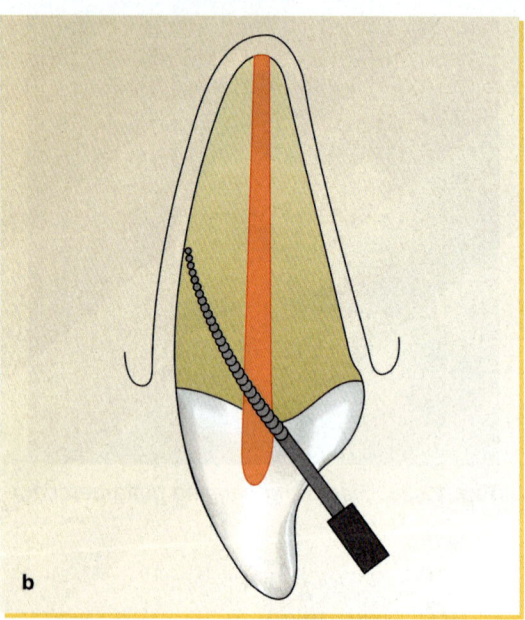

Fig. 12.41: *Perforation. (a) Cervical, (b) root*

Glossary

A

1. *Abfraction:* Wedge-shaped defects in the cervical region of tooth believed to be the result of tensile stresses concentrated in this area consequent to occlusal forces.
2. *Abrasion:* Lesions formed as a result of wearing away of tooth substance because of grinding, rubbing or scraping caused by external mechanical means like repeated contact of teeth with foreign objects.
3. *Abrasive cutting (grinding):* Use of bonded or coated abrasive instruments for removing surface layer of the substrate.
4. *Acid etch technique:* A procedure used to make the surface more reactive using an acidic solution (generally 37% phosphoric acid); improve the bond and marginal seal between resin and tooth.
5. *Acute caries:* Caries that is fast progressing and irreversible.
6. *Adherend:* Material to which adhesive is applied.
7. *Adhesion:* Force or intermolecular attraction that exists between the molecules of two unlike substances when placed in intimate contact with each other.
8. *Adhesive:* The substance added between two unlike substances to produce adhesion.
9. *Admixed alloy:* Mixture of two types of alloy particles, usually lathe cut and silver-copper eutectic.
10. *Advanced caries (cavitated caries):* Caries that has progressed to the dentino-enamel junction and is no longer reversible.
11. *Age hardening:* Hardening heat treatment for gold alloys; accomplished by aging the casting for 15–30 minutes at temperature between 200 and 450°C. Age hardening increases the proportional limit and hardness; whereas ductility is decreased.
12. *Alloy:* An alloy is a substance made by melting two or more elements together; at least one of them is metal.
13. *Amalgam blues:* Discoloration of tooth caused by leakage of corrosion products of amalgam restoration (usually occur where varnish is not applied).
14. *Amalgam substitutes:* Alloys containing components of amalgam but do not contain mercury, e.g. gallium alloys, mercury free direct filling alloys.
15. *Amalgam:* Amalgam is a mixture/alloy of mercury with one or more metals.

Generations of Amalgam

1st generation: 3 parts silver + 1 part tin (peritectic)

2nd generation: 1st generation + 4% copper + 1% zinc

3rd generation: 1st generation + silver copper eutectic

4th generation: 1st generation + 29% copper (high copper alloys)

5th generation: Quarternary alloy: Silver + tin + copper + indium

6th generation: Palladium, silver, copper eutectic + first, second and third generation

16. *Amalgapins:* A vertical post of amalgam anchored in the dentin.

17. *Anatomical tooth crown:* Portion of tooth covered with enamel.

18. *Anatomical tooth root:* Portion of tooth covered with cementum.

19. *Angle former:* It is a modified form of chisel. The primary cutting edge is sharpened at an angle to the axis of blade. Blade is beveled on the sides also, to form three cutting edges.

20. *Antibacterial composite:* Composite containing MDPB (methacryloxydecyl pyridinium bromide) with antibacterial properties.

21. *Anti-flux:* The material used to limit the action of flux, e.g. lead, graphite.

22. *Arrested caries:* Any carious lesion, usually an incipient, may become arrested, if there is a change in the oral environment. The arrested caries clinically appears as a dark brown pigmentation with smooth surface.

23. *Attrition:* Loss of tooth structure occurring as a result of frictional contact between opposing teeth.

24. *Automatrix:* It is a disposable system where band and retainer are constructed as one unit. It is primarily useful in patients who cannot tolerate retainers and in patients with partly erupted teeth.

25. *Axial wall:* Wall parallel to the long axis of tooth and facing the pulp.

B

1. *Back pressure porosity:* Porosity occurring in casting due to prevention of escapement of air due to bulk of investment.

2. *Backward caries:* When the spread of caries along dentinoenamel junction exceeds the caries in contagious enamel and caries extends back into enamel from DEJ.

3. *Base (cement base):*
   - High strength bases: Bases providing thermal protection to the pulp as well as mechanical support for the restoration, e.g. zinc phosphate, poly-carboxylate, glass ionomer cement.
   - Low strength bases having minimum strength and rigidity: Used mainly to act as barrier to irritating chemicals and therapeutic benefit to pulp, e.g. calcium hydroxide and zinc oxide eugenol.

4. *Base metal:* Metal elements that are chemically reactive to the air/environment, e.g. cobalt, chromium, etc.

5. *Beilby layer:* A microcrystalline surface layer that remains on cast restoration even after its final polishing.

6. *Bevel:* Any abrupt incline between two surfaces of prepared tooth or between cavosurface margins and cavity walls in prepared cavity.

Types of bevels and indications:

a. *Partial:* It involves part of enamel wall; indicated in direct filling gold.

b. *Short:* In involves entire enamel wall; indicated in cast gold inlays.

c. *Inverted:* It is given on the labial shoulder of metal ceramic crowns to effectively improve the esthetics at the margins.

d. *Reverse:* The bevel is placed at the dentinal portion of the cervical wall towards the axiopulpal line angle; indicated in cast gold inlays.

7. *Biological width:* Combined dimension of supra-alveolar gingival connective tissue and the junctional epithelium (0.97 mm + 1.07= 2.04 mm)

8. *Blade angle/tooth angle:* Angle between rake face and clearance face or land.

9. *Blade:* The projection on bur head.

10. *Blade:* Working end of cutting instrument.

11. *Bladed cutting:* Use of any instrument in blade like fashion.

12. *Buccal surface:* Surface of tooth facing the cheek (premolars and molars).
13. *Bur shape:* Contour or silhouette of bur head.
14. *Bur:* Rotary cutting instrument having two or more sharp edged blades with different shapes of cutting heads.
15. *Burn out:* Process of eliminating wax from the mold cavity and achieving thermal expansion.
16. *Burnishing:* It is a process in which smooth, rigid instrument is used for smoothening amalgam restoration that has become rough by carving.

C

1. *Carbon steel:* Alloy made up by addition of small percentage of carbon to iron [C– <2.0%, Fe:98.4 – 98.6%]
2. *Carving:* It is a process carried out to produce/simulate functional anatomy of any restoration.
3. *Cast:* A positive replica of several teeth or whole arch and their supporting structures.
4. *Cavit:* Premixed non-eugenol paste used for temporary restorations and also as cavity bases.
5. *Cavity liner:* Suspension of calcium hydroxide or zinc oxide in a volatile solvent, act as a barrier against the passage of irritants from cements or other restorative materials and to reduce sensitivity of freshly cut dentin (thickness– 0.5 mm).
6. *Cavity preparation:* Performance of all mechanical procedures required to remove the carious and affected tissues and to shape the remaining enamel and dentin so as to receive a biologically and mechanically sound restoration.
7. *Cavity varnish:* Solution of one or more resins which when applied on cavity walls, evaporates, leaving a thin film (usually 25 μ) that serves as a barrier between the restoration and the dentinal tubules; generally a natural gum (e.g.

copal, resin) or synthetic resin dissolved in organic solvent like alcohol, acetone or ether.

8. *Cavity:* Defect in enamel, dentin or cementum resulting from pathological processes, mostly dental caries.
9. *Cavosurface angle:* Angle formed at junction of cavity wall and the tooth surface.
10. *Cement:* Term used collectively for materials available as powder/liquid. When mixed, forms a paste that sets into a hard mass, can act as liner, base, luting agent and restorative material.
11. *Cementoenamel junction (CEJ):* The junction/union of enamel and cementum.
12. *Chelators:* A chelate refers to a compound with central metal surrounded by co-valently bonded atoms, ions or molecules called LIGANDS which possess additional bonds for chemical reaction.
13. *Chisel:* It is an instrument characterized by a blade that terminates in a cutting edge formed by a one sided bevel. Cutting edge of a chisel is at right angle to the shaft.
    Types of chisels:
    • Monoangle
    • Binangle
    • Triple angle
    • Straight
14. *Chroma:* It represents degree of saturation of a particular hue.
15. *Chronic caries:* Caries of slow onset and spread.
16. *Cingulum:* Lingual lobe of an anterior tooth making up the bulk of cervical 1/3rd of lingual surface.
17. *Circumferential tie:* Peripheral marginal anatomy of tooth preparation by which a favourable relationship is obtained between the casting and luting cement.
18. *Clearance angle:* Angle between clearance face and tooth.
    a. Primary clearance angle: Angle between land and work.

b. Secondary clearance angle: Angle between clearance face and work.

19. *Clearance face:* Surface of bur blade on trailing edge.

20. *Clinical tooth crown:* Portion of tooth exposed in oral cavity.

21. *Clinical tooth root:* Portion of root that is exposed in oral cavity.

22. *Colloidal silica:* Filler phase of composites.

23. *Coloring agents:* The materials used to change the hue of any restorative material.

24. *Complex cavity:* Cavity involving 3 or more surfaces, e.g. mesio-occlusodistal (MOD) cavity.

25. *Compomer:* Polyacid modified composites.

26. *Composite:* Compound of two or more distinctly different materials with properties that are superior or intermediate to those of individual constituent.

27. *Compound cavity:* Cavity involving 2 surfaces, e.g. bucco-occlusal or proximo-occlusal cavity.

28. *Concentricity:* Direct measurement of symmetry of the bur head.

29. *Condensable composites:* Based on PRIMM (Polymer Rigid Inorganic Matrix Material) concept; system of composites in which filler/inorganic phase is present as continuous network/scaffold instead of being incorporated as ground substance.

30. *Condensation:* It is a process by which the amalgam mix is compacted into prepared cavity to attain dense mass.

31. *Condenser:* Instruments used to condense the underlying restorative materials.

32. *Conditioning:* An alteration of tooth surface including the smear layer by either physical or chemical means with the objective of producing a surface capable of micromechanical and chemical bonding to the adhesive.

33. *Configuration factor (C-factor):* Ratio of bonded to unbonded surfaces in a composite restoration.

34. *Contact angle:* Angle formed by adhesive with adhered at their interface; a measure of wettability.

35. *Convenience form:* It is the shape or the form of cavity that allows adequate observation, accessibility and ease of operation in preparing and restoring the cavity.

36. *Conventional silver alloy:* Ag: 68–72%, Sn: 25–27%, Cu: 2–6%, Zn: 0–3%.

37. *Corrosion:* It is a process in which deterioration of a metal is caused by reaction with its environment.

38. *Coupling agent:* The material which is used to bind the matrix and filler phase in composites, e.g. γ-methacryloxy-propyltrimethoxysilane.

39. *Creep:* Time dependent plastic deformation of a material that occurs when it is subjected to a constant load near its melting point.

40. *Crosscuts:* Notches present on blade of instrument to obtain adequate cutting effectiveness at low and medium speeds.

41. *Crown:* Extra-coronal cast restoration in which all the cusps are covered.

42. *Cusp:* An elevation or mound on crown portion of tooth making up a divisional part of occlusal surface

43. *Custom tray:* A tray made for a specific patient according to his/her needs.

44. Cutting effectiveness of an instrument: Rate of removal of tooth in mm/min or mg/sec by that instrument.

45. *Cutting efficiency of an instrument:* Percentage of energy which produces cutting by that particular instrument.

D

1. *Delayed expansion:* It is the expansion occurring in zinc containing amalgam alloys due to contamination with moisture. It occurs within 3–5 days due to accumulation of hydrogen gas within the restoration.

2. *Dental caries:* Microbial disease of calcified tissues of teeth, characterized by demineralization of inorganic portion and destruction of organic substance of tooth.

3. *Dental casting investments:* A refractory material like silica, quartz or crystoballite added to dental plaster or stone; so that cast mold can be heated to high temperature.

4. *Dental impression:* The negative replica of tooth, teeth or its supporting structures.

5. *Dentin bonding agent:* Unfilled or semi-filled resins of low viscosity, consist of hydrophilic reactive group capable of bonding to dentin surface and hydrophobic methacrylate group capable of bonding to resin with spacer in between.

6. *Dentinal wall:* Portion of prepared external wall consisting of dentin; may contain retentive features.

7. *Dentinoenamel junction (DEJ):* The junction/union between enamel and dentin.

8. *Developmental groove:* A shallow groove on line between primary parts of crown or root.

9. *Die:* A die is the positive replica of single tooth.

10. *Die-stone (Type IV dental stone):* Improved stone used for making dies.

11. *Distal surface:* Proximal surface of tooth distant from medial line

12. *Distal wall:* Wall facing distal aspect of tooth.

13. *Double planed instruments:* These are the instruments in which the force is applied at a right angle to the plane of the blade and handle. These usually have a curved blade and are called double planed instruments.

14. *Double wedging:* Refers to insertion of two wedges; one from the lingual embrasure and the other from the buccal embrasure preferred in teeth with faciolingually wide proximal boxes.

E

1. *Eames technique (no squeeze cloth or minimal mercury technique):* The mercury alloy ratio according to this trituration technique is 1:1.

2. *Embrasures/Spillways:* These are V shaped spaces that originate at proximal contact area between adjacent teeth. These are facial, lingual, incisal/occlusal and gingival and these are continuous with each other as well as with interproximal spaces.

3. *Enameloplasty:* Process of conversion of shallow pit, fissure or groove into a rounded or saucered self cleansable area.

4. *Endodontics:* Endodontics is the branch of dentistry which deals with diagnosis, prognosis, treatment and prevention of diseases of pulp and periapical tissues.

5. *Erosions:* Lesions formed as a result of dissolution of tooth structure subsequent to chemical attack (endogenous or exogenous origin) or combined chemo-mechanical attack.

6. *Extension for prevention:* The phenomenon of including all susceptible fissures in the outline form. First suggested by Marshall Ebb and later adopted by Black.

7. *External line angle:* A line angle whose apex points away from tooth.

8. *External wall:* Surface of prepared cavity that extends onto exterior of tooth.

9. *Extra-coronal preparation:* The preparation that involves the external surfaces of tooth.

F

1. *Facial walls:* a. Labial: Wall facing the lips. b. Buccal: Wall facing the cheeks.

2. *Filler:* Particles which are added into composite resin matrix to improve its properties.

3. *Fissure:* Formed due to imperfect coalescence of developmental grooves during tooth development (more susceptible to caries).

4. *Floor/Seat of cavity:* Any cavity wall that is perpendicular to the forces directed occluso-gingivally, e.g. pulpal and gingival walls.

5. *Flow:* Property similar to creep but is applied for amorphous substances like waxes.

6. *Flowable composite:* Type of composites which contain 20–25% less filler particles and hence can easily flow due to their decreased viscosity.

7. *Flute (chip space):* Depressed areas present between uniformly spaced blades.

8. *Flux:* The material used for preventing, dissolving or removing the oxides formed on the surface of casting. Type of fluxes:

Type I: Protective fluxes: Prevent formation of oxides of metals, e.g. borates and boric acid.

Type II: Reduction fluxes: Reduce the oxides formed on surface of casting; used for noble metals, e.g. borates.

Type III: Dissolution fluxes: Remove the oxides by dissolving them; used for base metals, e.g. fluorides.

9. *Forward caries:* When caries cone in enamel is larger or at least of same size as in dentin.

10. *Fossa:* Irregular depression or concavity on tooth, cleansable.

G

1. *Gingival wall:* Wall facing gingiva and is perpendicular to the forces directed occlusogingivally.

2. *Giomer:* Pre-reacted glass-ionomer particles added to composites.

3. *Glass cermet (cermet):* Glass ionomer powder particles are sintered with metal (silver/tin/palladium) particle in the ratio of 7:1.

4. *Gold alloy:* Alloy of gold with other metals. It is of 4 types:

Type I: Gold is 80–90% (87%)
Type II: Gold is 75–80% (76%)
Type III: Gold is 70–75% (70%)
Type IV: Gold is 60–70% (66%)

5. *Green strength:* Wet strength of gypsum products.

6. *Green shrinkage:* A volumetric contraction which accompanies the drying process due to loss of alcohol and water which reduces the size of the mold.

7. *Grooves:* Secondary retentive devices; given for cast restorations.

8. *Grooving:* Restoring the depth of development grooves which have been reduced by occlusal wear.

9. *Guards:* Finger positions of hand, opposite the one using the instrument to steady the parts being operated on and to protect them from injury in case the instrument slips.

H

1. *Hand cutting instruments:* Instruments which are used with manual force.

2. *High copper amalgam:* Amalgam alloys containing more than 6% (5–30%) of copper content.

3. *Hue:* Specific colour produced by specific wavelength of light, e.g. red, green, yellow etc.

4. *Hybrid layer:* Dentin bonding, micro-mechanical attachment between resin and demineralized and primed surface layer of intertubular dentin.

I

1. *Impression:* Negative replica of any object.

2. *Incipient caries (initial caries):* Evident as white opaque area on surface of enamel.

3. *Indirect method of wax pattern preparation:* The method of wax pattern preparation in which pattern is prepared on the die.

4. *Inlay casting wax:* Wax used to make pattern for inlays.

5. *Inlay:* An intracoronal cast restoration designed mainly to restore occlusal/proximal surface(s) of posterior teeth without involving the cusps.

6. *Internal line angle:* An angle whose apex points into the tooth.

7. *Intracoronal cavity preparation:* Cavity that is prepared in the interior of tooth.

L

1. *Labial surface:* Surface of tooth (anterior teeth) facing lips.
2. *Land:* The plane surface immediately following the cutting edge is called the land.
3. *Line angle:* The junction of two surfaces along a definite line.
4. *Lingual surfaces:* The surfaces of teeth facing tongue.
5. *Lingual wall:* Wall of prepared cavity facing the tongue.
6. *Lobe:* Primary sections of formation of the development of crown of tooth.
7. *Locks:* Given in the proximal boxes; 0.2–0.3 mm wide and 0.5 mm in depth for silver amalgam restorations.
8. *Low copper amalgam:* Amalgam alloys containing less than 6% copper content.
9. *Ligand:* Ion or a molecule attached to a metal atom by coordinate bonding.

M

1. *Mamelons:* Rounded protuberances on the incisal ridges of newly erupted permanent incisor teeth (generally three).
2. *Matricing:* Procedure whereby temporary wall is created opposite to axial walls and surrounding areas of tooth structure that was lost during preparation.
3. *Matrix retainers:* Gadgets used to retain matrix band in position.
4. *Matrix:* A device used to contour a restoration to simulate that of tooth configuration.
5. *Mesial surface:* The surface of tooth facing medial line.
6. *Mesial wall:* Wall of prepared cavity facing mesial aspect of tooth.
7. *Microleakage:* The clinically undetectable passage of bacteria and bacterial products, fluids, molecules or ions from the oral environment along the gaps present in cavity-restoration interface.
8. *Microporosity:* Porosity occurring in casting due to rapid solidification shrinkage.
9. *Miracle mix:* A modified form of glass ionomer cement in which silver-tin alloy powder is added to GIC powder.
10. *Mulling:* It is a process by which amalgam mix is given a cohesive form by taking mix in hand and rubbing between fingers.

N

1. *Nib:* Working end of non-cutting instrument (also called face).
2. *Noble metals:* Metals which does not easily react to environment, e.g. gold, silver, platinum, palladium, etc.

O

1. *Oblique ridge:* Ridge formed by joining the triangular ridge of mesiolingual and distobuccal cusps of maxillary first permanent molar; crosses the occlusal surface obliquely.
2. *Occlusal surfaces:* Surfaces of posterior teeth which come in contact with those of opposing arch during maximum intercuspation.
3. *Onlay:* Combination of intracoronal and extracoronal cast restoration when one or more cusps are covered and not all.
4. *Operative dentistry:* The branch of dentistry which deals with diagnosis, prognosis, treatment and prevention of defects of teeth, restoring them to their form, function and esthetics, thereby maintaining stomatognathic system.
5. *Outline form:* Area of tooth surface or the enamel margin to be included in the prepared cavity.
6. *Overbite:* Vertical distance from incisal edges of maxillary anterior to incisal edges of mandibular anteriors (2.0–3.0 mm).
7. *Overjet:* Horizontal distance between labial surface of mandibular anteriors and lingual surfaces of maxillary anteriors (2.0–3.0 mm).

P

1. *Palatal surfaces:* Surfaces of teeth facing palate (maxillary teeth).
2. *Palatal wall:* Wall of prepared cavity facing palate.
3. *Pickling:* The casting is cleaned with 50% hydrochloric acid or 50% sulphuric acid to remove discoloration of gold alloys after casting.
4. *Piggy back wedging:* Method of wedge placement; useful in gingival recession. A smaller second wedge is placed on first to prevent gingival overhanging.
5. *Pit and fissure caries:* Caries beginning in pits and fissures of teeth.
6. *Pit:* Small pin point depressions located at the terminal or junction of developmental grooves.
7. *Point angle:* The junction of three surfaces at a point, e.g. axio-faciopulpal point angle.
8. *Primary flare:* The flaring of lingual wall and buccal wall of proximal box from the axial wall (axiolingual and axiofacial line angles respectively) to the proximal cavosurface margins is known as primary flare.
9. *Primer:* Adhesion promoting agents; used to promote the diffusion of resin into moist, demineralized dentin so as to achieve complete resin penetration.
10. *PRIMM:* Polymer rigid inorganic matrix material; concept used for condensable (packable) composites.
11. *Proximal surfaces:* Surfaces of teeth facing adjoining teeth in same dental arch.
12. *Pulpal wall:* Wall facing pulp and perpendicular to the long axis of tooth.

Q

1. *Qualitative violation of crevice:* When there is irritation of crevice due to poor adaptation and roughness of margins of restoration.

2. *Quantitative violation of crevice:* When excessive material is placed in crevice, e.g. overhanging margins of restoration.
3. *Quaternary alloys:* Single composition containing silver, copper, tin and indium.

R

1. *Radial clearance:* If the clearance face is curved, it is known as radial clearance.
2. *Radial line:* Line connecting the centre of bur and blade.
3. *Rake angle:* Angle between rake face and radial line.
4. *Rake face:* Surface of bur blade on the leading edge.
5. *Removal of remaining carious dentin:* Elimination of any infected carious tooth structure or faulty restoration left in cavity preparation.
6. *Residual caries:* Caries that remain even after cavity preparation is completed.
7. *Resin matrix:* The continuous phase of resin materials in which fillers are added viz. Bis-GMA, TEGDMA, UDMA, etc.
8. *Resin modified glass ionomer cement:* Modified form of GIC in which resins, such as Bis-GMA, TEGDMA are added to powder and HEMA to liquid. Sets by light exposure as well as chemical reaction.
9. *Resistance form:* The shape and configuration of the cavity that best enables the restoration and the tooth to withstand occlusal forces without fracture.
10. *Rests:* Rests are used to steady hand during operative procedures.
11. *Retention form:* The shape and configuration of cavity that enable the restoration to be retained in that cavity under all types of stresses.
12. *Ridge:* A linear elevation on tooth surface; named according to location (buccal, cervical, incisal ridge, etc.).
13. *Root caries (senile caries):* Caries on the roots of teeth that have been exposed to oral environment.

14. *Rotary cutting instruments:* Group of instruments that turn on an axis to perform work, such as cutting, abrading, burnishing, finishing or polishing tooth tissues or restoration.

15. *Run out:* Dynamic measurement of maximum displacement of bur head while bur runs [0.023 mm].

S

1. *Sandwich technique (Bilayered restorations):* A technique for restoring a tooth in which glass ionomer cement is used as liner and cavity is filled with composite resin.

2. *Saturation:* Amount of color per unit area of an object.

3. *Secondary caries (recurrent caries):* Caries beginning around or beneath a restoration.

4. *Secondary flare:* Beveling the cavosurface margins of primary flare (given in gold inlays).

5. *Sensitivity:* Ability of a test to correctly identify those patients with the disease.

6. *Simple cavity:* Cavity in which only one surface of tooth is involved.

7. *Single composition alloy (all in one alloy):* Each particle of this alloy has same chemical composition.

8. *Skirts:* Extensions of proximal box at line angles of tooth or even away from it (given in cast restoration).

9. *Slots (horizontal groove):* 1.0–1.5 mm deep, box shaped preparations given along the occlusal or gingival walls.

10. *Smear layer:* A protein rich film along with dentinal shavings and debris found on the grounded tooth surface.

11. *Smooth surface caries:* Caries beginning on the smooth surfaces.

12. *Soft steel:* Steel containing 0.25% or less carbon.

13. *Softening heat treatment (solution heat treatment):* For gold alloys: casting is heated for 10 minutes at 700°C and immediately quenched in water; increases ductility and softens the casting.

14. *Specificity:* Ability of a test to correctly identify those patients without the disease.

15. *Spheroiding:* Reducing the prematurities while restoring original tooth contour.

16. *Sprue former:* Made up of wax, plastic or hollow metal, act as a channel for entry of molten alloy during casting and elimination of wax during burnout.

17. *Stainless steel:* Carbon: 0.2–1.2%, chromium: 18%, iron: 81–81.4%

18. *Step:* Auxiliary extension of main cavity on adjoining surface.

19. *Strain hardening:* Hardening treatment for cobalt chromium alloys, increases hardness and strength and decreases ductility.

20. *Subpulpal wall:* When the roof of pulp chamber is removed, the floor of pulp chamber left behind is referred to as subpulpal wall.

21. *Subsurface porosity (pinhole porosity):* Spherical voids in casting, due to rapid entry of alloy in mold.

22. *Suck back porosity (shrink spot porosity):* Porosity occurring in casting due to shrinkage of molten alloy on cooling; irregular voids in casting.

23. *Sulcus:* Long depression or valley in surface of tooth between cusps and ridges.

T

1. *Tarnish:* The surface discoloration of a metal or the slight loss/alteration of surface finish/polish.

2. *Ternary alloys:* Single composition alloys containing silver, tin and copper.

3. *Tofflemire matrix:* A band retainer, available in two forms – straight and contra-angled, and is used for MOD and C-II restorations.

4. *Transverse ridge:* Formed by union of buccal and lingual triangular ridge; crossing the occlusal surface of posterior tooth transversely, e.g. in permanent mandibular first molar.

5. *Triangular ridge:* Ridges descending from cusp tips of posterior teeth towards the central portion of tooth and have slopes of each side inclined such that they resemble two sides of triangle; named according to the cusp involved, e.g. triangular ridge of buccal cusp of maxillary first premolar.

6. *Trituration:* The process of mixing alloy powder with mercury.

7. *Twist drill:* A device which is used to prepare pin holes.

V

1. *Value:* The lightness or darkness of an object.

2. *Veneers:* Wafer thin shells of tooth colored materials like composite, porcelains, etc. that are bonded on the front side of teeth for cosmetic improvement of teeth.

W

1. *Wall:* Any surface of prepared cavity.
2. *Wedge wedging:* Method of wedge placement for maxillary first premolar; a second wedge is inserted from occlusal side between the first wedge and band.
3. *Wedge:* Component of matrix system used to prevent overhanging of the restorations (triangular/trapezoidal shape).

Z

1. *Zinc containing amalgam:* Amalgam alloy containing more than 0.01% of zinc.
2. *Zinc free amalgam:* Amalgam alloy containing less than 0.01% of zinc.

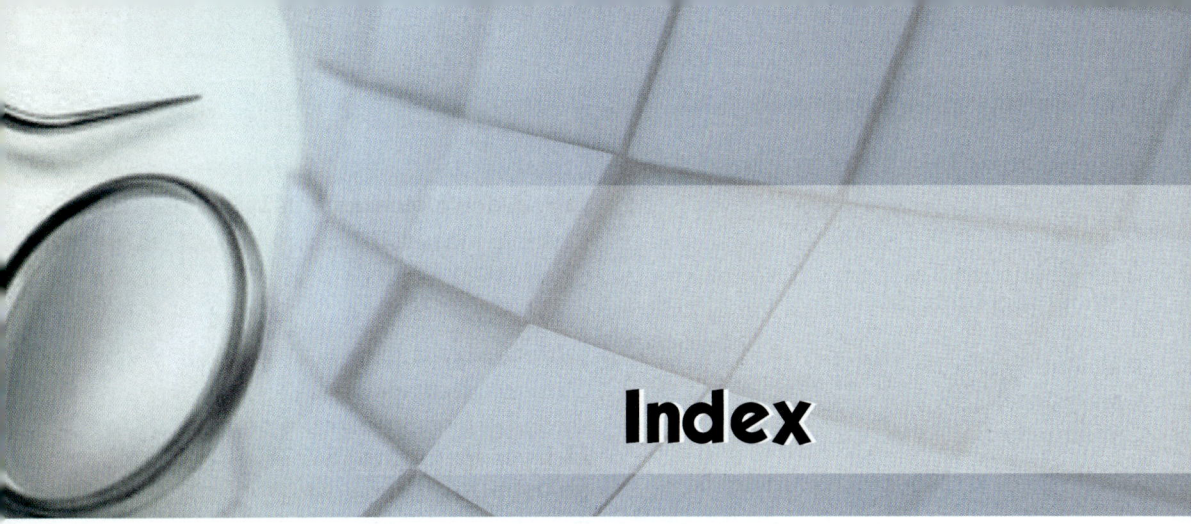

Index